DUFF

MRI of the Spine

Second Edition

The LWW MRI Teaching File Series

SERIES EDITORS

Robert B. Lufkin
William G. Bradley, Jr.
Michael Brant-Zawadzki

MRI of the Brain I

Michael Brant-Zawadzki and William G. Bradley, Jr., Editors

MRI of the Brain II

William G. Bradley, Jr. and Michael Brant-Zawadzki, Editors

MRI of the Spine

Jeffrey S. Ross, Author

MRI of the Head and Neck

Robert B. Lufkin, Editor

MRI of the Musculoskeletal System

Minnie Pathria and Karence Chan, Editors

Pediatric MRI

Rosalind B. Dietrich, Editor

The LWW MRI Teaching File Series

MRI of the Spine

Second Edition

Editor

JEFFREY S. ROSS, M.D.

Head of Research and Staff Neuroradiologist
Department of Radiology
Cleveland Clinic Foundation
Cleveland, Ohio

LIPPINCOTT WILLIAMS & WILKINS
A **Wolters Kluwer** Company
Philadelphia · Baltimore · New York · London
Buenos Aires · Hong Kong · Sydney · Tokyo

Acquisitions Editor: Joyce-Rachel John
Developmental Editor: Anjou K. Dargar
Production Editor: Karen Tates-Denton
Manufacturing Manager: Tim Reynolds
Cover Designer: David Levy
Compositor: Maryland Composition
Printer: Maple Press

© 2000 by LIPPINCOTT WILLIAMS & WILKINS
530 Walnut Street
Philadelphia, PA 19106-3780 USA
LWW.com

Printed in the USA

Library of Congress Cataloging-in-Publication Data
MRI of the spine / editor, Jeffrey S. Ross.
     p. ; cm.—(The LWW MRI teaching file)
    Includes bibliographical references and index.
    ISBN 0-7817-2528-3
     1. Spine—Magnetic resonance imaging. 2. Spine—Diseases—Diagnosis. 3. Magnetic resonance imaging. I. Ross, Jeffrey S. (Jeffrey Stuart) II. Series.
    [DNLM: 1. Spinal Diseases—diagnosis. 2. Magnetic Resonance Imaging. WE 725
M9392   2000]
RD768.M752   2000
617.5'607548—dc21

                                                   99-048216

10 9 8 7 6 5 4 3 2 1

DEDICATION

My son, if you accept my words
  and store up my commands within you,
turning your ear to wisdom
  and applying your heart to understanding,
and if you call out for insight
  and cry aloud for understanding,
and if you look for it as for silver
  and search for it as for hidden treasure,
then you will understand the fear of the LORD
  and find the knowledge of God.
For the LORD gives wisdom,
  and from his mouth come knowledge and understanding.
                                        Proverbs 2:1–6

CONTENTS

PREFACE

The past ten years have witnessed a revolution in the diagnosis and management of spinal disorders. Magnetic resonance (MR) imaging has quickly emerged as the study of choice for virtually all disorders of the spine, with computed tomography (CT) continuing to play an important, but ancillary role. With the inherent contrast sensitivity and multiplanar imaging capability of MR, the morphology of the vertebrae, intervertebral disk, epidural space, cord, and roots can be visualized with striking clarity. Contrast administration allows definition of abnormal vessels, leptomeninges, and disrupted blood-cord barrier.

It must always be remembered, however, that the body has a limited range of responses to an apparently infinite variety of insults from infectious, inflammatory, traumatic, and neoplastic entities. While providing the single correct diagnosis is the goal, the images are often sensitive but not specific, and a logical pathologic differential diagnosis must be given. Further, as more experience has been gained, it has become clear that many morphologic derangements can be demonstrated in asymptomatic individuals, which further complicates the concept of "abnormality". These facts emphasize the central importance of the clinical evaluation in the work-up of patients with spine disorders.

In this book a wide variety of spinal disorders are presented, extending from the mundane to the esoteric. For each case, a brief statement of clinical presentation is given, with the imaging findings and a discussion of the pathology. This is not an all-inclusive collection, but rather a broad case mix to show patterns of disease. The vast bulk of the cases have been collected from routine reading sessions. Low field and high field images have been included in the collection, and the technical parameters have been kept to a minimum.

I hope you find these cases challenging and informative. Ultimately, I hope this translates into improved diagnoses and better patient management.

Jeffrey S. Ross, M.D.

The LWW MRI Teaching File Series

MRI of the Spine

Second Edition

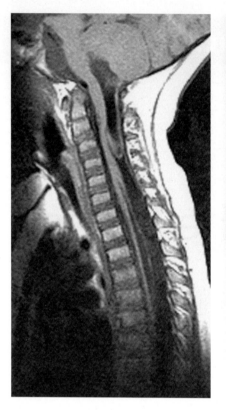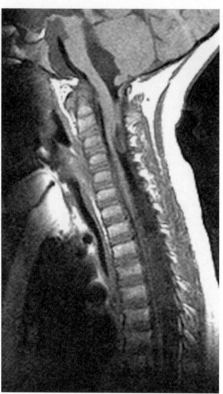

FIGURE 1.1   **FIGURE 1.2**

HISTORY

A 1-year-old with a history of hydrocephalus.

FINDINGS

Two sagittal T1-weighted images demonstrate marked descent of the cerebellar tonsils below the level of the foramen magnum. As there is an elongated and distorted fourth ventricle, which extends into the upper cervical canal. There is linear CSF signal intensity within the cervical cord more inferiorly reflecting syrinx. The superior aspect of the images shows a small posterior fossa with a vertically oriented straight sinus.

DIAGNOSIS

Chiari II malformation with cervical syrinx.

DISCUSSION

Professor Hans Chiari described the malformation named after him in 1896 (type II), consisting of caudal descent of the cerebellar vermis, fourth ventricle, and lower brain stem that is almost always seen in conjunction with a myelomeningocele. The type I lesion was described in 1891 and is characterized by caudal descent of the cerebellar tonsils. Type III Chiari malformation is an occipital encephalocele of the cerebellum, whereas the type IV lesion was cerebellar hypoplasia (and not herniation). Clinical symptoms in Chiari II are varied, but one-third of myelomeningocele patients will develop brain stem symptoms by 5 years of age. Apnea, feeding, and swallowing difficulties are also prevalent. Older children are likely to develop cord or cerebellar symptoms with pain, sensory loss, and ataxia. Older children can also present with weakness or spasticity.

Hydrosyringomyelia describes the cavitation of the spinal cord. Syringes are seen in approximately 50% to 75% of Chiari I malformations and in 50% to 90% of Chiari II malformations. The terms *syringomyelia* and *hydromyelia* refer to different conditions: In syringomyelia the lining is glial cells, and in hydromyelia the lining is ependymal cells, which is in continuity with the central canal. The combined word *syringohydromyelia* may also be used, given our inability to distinguish these types in most cases. When in doubt, just say *syrinx*. Multiple theories have been offered to explain the pathophysiology that produces cystic cavitation of the spinal cord. W.J. Gardner initially attempted to explain the mechanism behind syrinx cavities from work in treating patients with a Chiari malformation, maintaining that in such patients normal CSF egress from the fourth ventricle is prevented by congenital obstruction of the foramina of Magendie and Luschka. As a result, systolic CSF pressure pulsations generated by the choroid plexus are transmitted to the central canal of the cord via the obex of the fourth ventricle. Thus the syrinx consists of a dilated central canal and/or diverticula of the central canal that extend by dissecting along the spinal cord fiber tracts. This theory fails to explain such cavities in patients whose foramina of the fourth ventricle are patent, who have no hindbrain malformations, and in whom the syrinx and fourth ventricle do not communicate. Williams modified the Gardner theory by considering intracranial and spinal venous and CSF pressure shifts. He maintained that coughing, sneezing, and Valsalva maneuvers can increase intraspinal venous distention, thus raising intraspinal CSF pressures. In the presence of partial spinal block (e.g., at the foramen magnum in Chiari malformation) a ball-valve phenomenon exists. When CSF pressure is increased below the lesion, fluid is forced temporarily above the point of obstruction. When venous pressure returns to normal, CSF pressure remains elevated above the site of block, which then forces fluid into the central canal below the block until the pressures equalize. Ball and Dayan have questioned these theories on other grounds. They calculated the pulse pressure wave transmitted to the cord substance under the circumstances just described to be such that it would not likely produce cord cavitation. Instead, they maintained, CSF under pressure secondary to subarachnoid obstruction would track into the spinal cord by way of the Virchow-Robin spaces. Subsequently, small collections of CSF would coalesce to form larger syrinx cavities that might or might not connect to the central canal. Quencer et al. have invoked an analogous theory to explain the development of syrinx cavities in patients with intradural extramedullary neoplasms. They maintain that longstanding compression, secondary to such mass lesions, results in permanent enlargement or microcystic change of the perivascular space, which then predisposes to the development of syrinx cavities.

Despite the lack of a comprehensive theory on the pathogenesis of spinal cord cystic cavities, a unifying theme among all the hypotheses put forth to date is the presence of dissecting and moving CSF shifts. This is important because such CSF motion may have significant impact on the MR imaging appearance of the syrinx cavity.

BIBLIOGRAPHY

Ball MJ, Dayan AD. Pathogenesis of syringomyelia. *Lancet* 1972;2:799–801.

Barnes PD, Brody JD, Jaramillo D, et al. Atypical idiopathic scoliosis: MR imaging evaluation. *Radiology* 1993;186: 247–253.

Cai C, Oakes WJ. Hindbrain herniation syndromes: the Chiari malformations (I and II). *Semin Pediatr Neurol* 1997;4: 179–191.

Gardner WJ. Hydrodynamic mechanism of syringomyelia—its relationship to myelocele. *J Neurol Neurosurg Psychiatry* 1965;28:247–259.

Gardner LW, Angel J. The mechanism of syringomyelia and its surgical connection. *Clin Neurosurg* 1975;6:131–140.

Milhorat TH, Capocelli ALJ, Anzil AP, et al. Pathological basis of spinal cord cavitation in syringomyelia: analysis of 105 autopsy cases. *J Neurosurg* 1995;82:802–812.

Pillay PK, Awad IA, Little JR, et al. Surgical management of syringomyelia: a five-year experience in the era of magnetic resonance imaging. *Neurol Res* 1991;13:3–9.

Quencer RM, el Gammal T, Cohen G. Syringomyelia associated with intradural extramedullary masses of the spinal canal. *Am J Neuroradiol* 1986;7:143–148.

Vaquero J, Martinez R, Arias A. Syringomyelia-Chiari complex: magnetic resonance imaging and clinical evaluation of surgical treatment. *J Neurosurg* 1990;73:64–68.

Williams B. Current concepts in syringomyelia. *Br J Hosp Med* 1970;4:331–342.

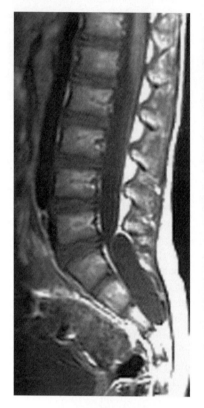

FIGURE 2.1

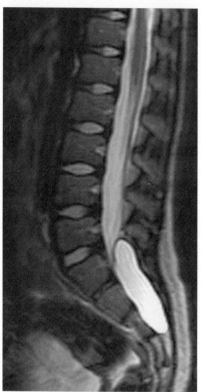

FIGURE 2.2

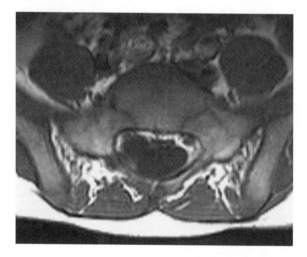

FIGURE 2.3

HISTORY

A 9-year-old with urinary incontinence.

FINDINGS

Sagittal T1-weighted, sagittal T2-weighted, and axial T1-weighted images of the lumbar spine show a well-defined mass tracking CSF signal intensity involving the sacral canal. This shows a capped superior and inferior margin, with evidence of bony expansion and remodeling of the posterior elements. The exiting roots appear displaced around the lesion on the axial T1-weighted image. The conus is normal in position, and the rest of the vertebral bodies and posterior elements are normal.

DIAGNOSIS

Sacral meningeal cyst, type I.

DISCUSSION

Nabors et al. have clarified the confusing array of terms for spinal meningeal cysts. Spinal meningeal cysts are congenital diverticula of the dural sac, root sheaths, or arachnoid that may be classified into three major groups. The first include extradural cysts without spinal nerve roots (type I); the second, extradural cysts with spinal nerve roots (type II); and the third, intradural cysts (type III). Type I—extradural meningeal cysts without roots—consists of diverticula that maintain contact with the thecal sac by a narrow ostium. This term includes extradural cysts, pouches, and diverticula as well as the so-called occult intrasacral meningoceles. Sacral type I cysts are found in adults and are connected to the tip of the caudal thecal sac by a pedicle.

Type II meningeal cysts with nerve roots are extradural lesions, previously called *Tarlov cysts, perineural cysts,* or *nerve root diverticula.* These are generally seen as multiple incidental lesions but are occasionally associated with radiculopathy or incontinence. Type III meningeal cysts are intradural lesions most commonly found on the posterior subarachnoid space and have been called *arachnoid diverticula* or *arachnoid cysts.* These are lined by a single layer of normal arachnoid cells and are filled with CSF. Dural ectasia associated with such entities as neurofibromatosis, Marfan's syndrome, and Ehlers-Danlos syndrome can occasionally mimic a meningeal cyst and should be considered in the appropriate clinical context.

BIBLIOGRAPHY

Nabors MW, Pait TG, Byrd EB, et al. Updated assessment and current classification of spinal meningeal cysts. *J Neurosurg* 1988;68:366–377.

Kronborg O. Extradural spinal cysts: a literature survey and a case of multiple extradural cysts. *Dan Med Bull* 1967;14: 46–48.

Rohrer DC, Burchiel KJ, Gruber DP. Intraspinal extradural meningeal cyst demonstrating ball-valve mechanism of formation: case report. *J Neurosurg* 1993;78:122–125.

Rothman RH, Jacobs SR, Appleman W. Spinal extradural cysts: a report of five cases. *Clin Orthop* 1970;71:186–192.

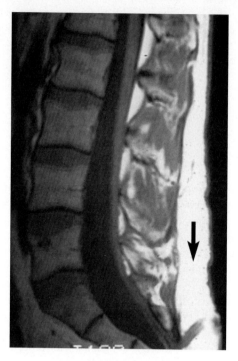

FIGURE 3.1

HISTORY

A 20-year-old with history of meningitis, and hairy patch on low back.

FINDINGS

Sagittal T1-weighted image shows that linear area of soft-tissue signal intensity over the S3 segment extending toward the thecal sac (*arrow*). This soft-tissue signal is contiguous with the intrathecal filum terminale in the midline. The conus is abnormal, being indistinct and showing a thickened filum extending down into the sacral segments.

DIAGNOSIS

Dermal sinus with tethered cord.

DISCUSSION

Dorsal dermal sinus is a midline sinus tract lined by epithelium that extends inward from the skin surface for a variable distance. It may terminate in the subcutaneous tissues or extend deeper to communicate with the conus and cord. This is thought to arise from a focal or incomplete disjunction of the cutaneous ectoderm from the neural ecto-derm. The epithelium lining the tract may also produce a dermoid or epidermoid in 30% to 50% of cases.

Dorsal dermal sinus occurs most frequently in the sacrococcygeal region. Above this level, it will extend into the spinal canal or cord. The sinus is seen in equal frequencies in boys and girls. A hypopigmented patch or capillary angioma is usually associated with the skin dimple. Patients can present with infection or signs of cord or nerve recompression from the intradural dermoid or epidermoid. The intraspinal portion of the tract may be very difficult to visualize with MR. The extraspinal portion can also be difficult, given the patient positioning and the high signal intensity typically associated with the dorsal subcutaneous tissues close to the surface coil. Attention to window and level settings is critical for finding these subtle tracts.

BIBLIOGRAPHY

Barkovich AJ, Edwards Ms, Cogen PH. MR evaluation of spinal dermal sinus tracts in children. *Am J Neuroradiol* 1991;12:123–129.

Goske MJ, Modic MT, Yu S. Pediatric spine: normal anatomy and spinal dysraphism. In: Modic MT, Masaryk TJ, Ross JS, eds. *Magnetic resonance imaging of the spine.* St Louis: Mosby-Year Book, 1994.

Rindahl MA, Colletti PM, Zee CS, et al. Magnetic resonance imaging of pediatric spinal dysraphism. *Maga Reson Imaging* 1989;7:217–224.

Wright RL. Congenital dermal sinuses. *Prog Neurol Surg* 1971;4:175–191.

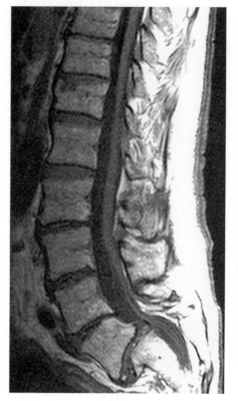

FIGURE 4.1

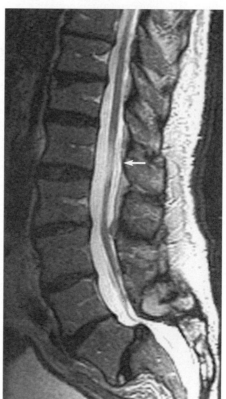

FIGURE 4.2

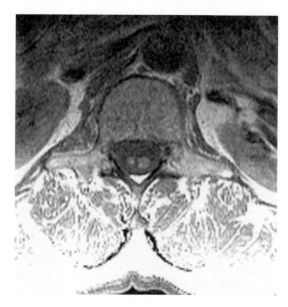

FIGURE 4.3

HISTORY

A 34-year-old with back pain.

FINDINGS

Sagittal T1-weighted (Fig. 4.1) and sagittal T2-weighted (Fig. 4.2) images of the lumbar spine show an indistinct conus and a thickened filum terminale consistent with tethering. There is abnormal increase signal on the sagittal T2-weighted images following the course of the cauda equina and filum terminale at the L1–2 level (*arrow*). At this level on the axial T1-weighted image (Fig. 4.3), two rounded soft-tissue signals are seen due to the presence of two hemicords. Of incidental note is marked and diffuse degenerative disk disease and an old compression fracture of the T12 body.

DIAGNOSIS

Diastematomyelia (single dural investment).

DISCUSSION

Diastematomyelia (DSM) is a form of spinal dysraphism characterized by partial or complete sagittal cleft of one or more segments of the spinal cord, conus medullaris, or filum terminale. Two hemicords are produced with one central canal, one dorsal horn, and one ventral horn, each supplying the ipsilateral nerve roots. The term *diastematomyelia* refers to the clefting of the cord, not necessarily the fibrous or bony spur. There is a female predominance of 80% to 94% of cases of DSM. The bone spur has a variable appearance, as it is formed in cartilage and ossifies variably through life. Most spurs form in the lower thoracic and lumbar spine. Ninety-one percent of hemicords will reunite. Coronal imaging often best demonstrates the cleft, which may be missed on sagittal imaging. The presumed etiology is an early splitting of the notocord, which will induce the overlying ectoderm to form neuroectoderm. The two sites of neuroectoderm formation thus give rise to two hemicords. Since the notocord is also responsible for vertebral body development, associated vertebral body and posterior element anomalies are extremely common. The pathognomonic bone finding for DSM is intersegmental laminar fusion.

A single dural investiture as shown in this case occurs in approximately 50% of cases. A single dura implies that no spur is present. This type of DSM may be seen incidentally in adults, since without a spur there is no cause for cord tethering. The increased signal on the sagittal T2-weighted image is due to partial volume effects from the CSF in between the two hemicords.

BIBLIOGRAPHY

Byrd SE, Darling CF, McLone DG. Developmental disorders of the pediatric spine. *Radiol Clin North Am* 1991;29: 711–752.

Goske MJ, Modic MT, Yu S. Pediatric spine: normal anatomy and spinal dysraphism. In: Modic MT, Masaryk TJ, Ross JS, eds. *Magnetic resonance imaging of the spine.* St Louis: Mosby-Year Book, 1994.

Pang D, Hoffman HJ, Rekate HL. Split cord malformation. Part II: clinical syndrome.

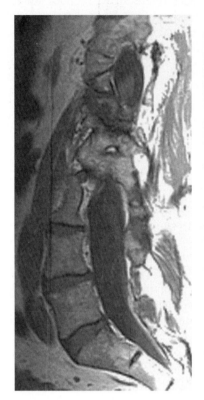

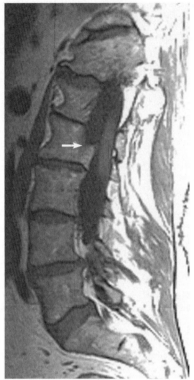

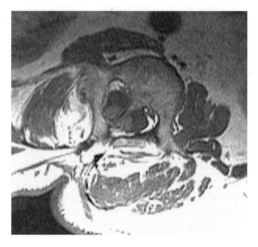

FIGURE 5.1   **FIGURE 5.2**   **FIGURE 5.3**

HISTORY

A 16-year-old with scoliosis and back pain.

FINDINGS

Sagittal (Figs. 5.1, 5.2) and axial (Fig. 5.3) T1-weighted images show a complex scoliosis of the thoracolumbar junction, and evidence of vertebral segmentation anomalies. There is fusion of the laminae at the L1–2 level and a bony spur arising off the posterior inferior aspect of the L2 body (*arrow*). Closer inspection of this spur on the axial image shows that the spur extends posteriorly in the midline and divides the dura into two separate areas, each with its own hemicord.

DIAGNOSIS

Diastematomyelia with spur.

DISCUSSION

Diastematomyelia is a sagittal splitting of the spinal cord into two segments. There are two general types. In approximately 50% of cases, the dural tube is undivided, in that both hemicords are contained by a single dural investiture.

Clinical findings tend to be rare in this group, and surgery is not indicated because there is no cord tethering and no spur. In the other half, as in this case, there is complete or partial splitting of the dural sac by a fibrous, cartilaginous, or bony spur, which causes tethering of the cord. The hemicords can be asymmetric in size, and there can be a syrinx in one cord and not the other. In more than 90% of the cases the split cord will reunite inferior to the location of the spur. Imaging is more complicated because of the association of the spinal segmentation and vertebral body anomalies, as well as the severe presence of scoliosis. Coronal imaging can be very helpful in this regard to define the site of the diastematomyelia and the positioning of the spur. Sagittal imaging alone is not adequate to exclude the diagnosis, since the vertically oriented hemicords may be missed due to partial volume effects.

BIBLIOGRAPHY

Byrd SE, Darling CF, McLone DG. Developmental disorders of the pediatric spine. *Radiol Clin North Am* 1991;29: 711–752.

Goske MJ, Modic MT, Yu S. Pediatric spine: normal anatomy and spinal dysraphism. In: Modic MT, Masaryk TJ, Ross JS, eds. *Magnetic resonance imaging of the spine.* St Louis: Mosby-Year Book, 1994.

Pang D, Hoffman HJ, Rekate HL. Split cord malformation. Part II: clinical syndrome. *Neurosurgery* 1992;31:481–500.

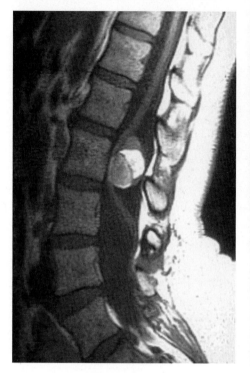

FIGURE 6.1

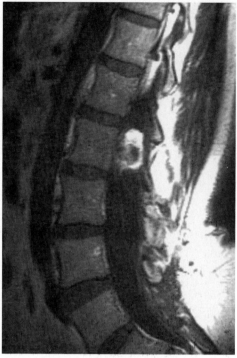

FIGURE 6.2

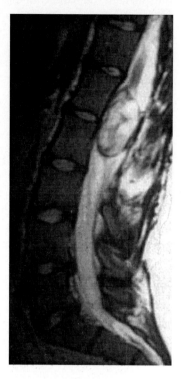

FIGURE 6.3

HISTORY

A 20-year-old with constipation.

FINDINGS

Sagittal T1-weighted images (Figs. 6.1, 6.2) and the sagittal T2-weighted image (Fig. 6.3) show a complex mass of mixed signal intensity on both T1- and T2-weighted sequences at the L2 level. The mass appears intradural and displaces the conus and cauda equina anteriorly around the lesion. There is evidence of dorsal dysraphism at the L3 through the L5 levels. The mass shows a strikingly high signal on the T1-weighted images.

DIAGNOSIS

Epidermoid tumor.

DISCUSSION

Intradural extramedullary tumors in children include neurofibromas, lipomas, dermoids, epidermoids, and teratomas. Epidermoid tumors should be considered or associated with a dermal sinus that must be carefully looked for within the dorsal soft tissues. Acquired epidermoids can re-

sult from implantation of epidermoid iatrogenically by spinal needles. It has been estimated that 40% of intraspinal epidermoids are iatrogenic in origin. Clinical presentation is variable and includes back pain, radiculopathy, alteration of gait, and difficulty in walking.

BIBLIOGRAPHY

Caro PA, Marks HG, Keret D, et al. Intraspinal epidermoid tumors in children: problems in recognition and imaging techniques for diagnosis. *J Pediatr Orthop* 1991;11:288–293.

Roeder MB, Bazan C, Jinkins JR. Ruptured spinal dermoid cyst with chemical arachnoiditis and disseminated intracranial lipid droplets. *Neuroradiology* 1995;37:146–147.

Toro VE, Lacy C, Binet EF. MRI of iatrogenic spinal epidermoid tumor. *J Comput Assist Tomogr* 1993;17:970–972.

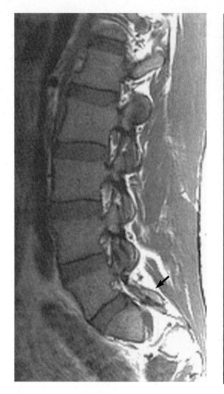

FIGURE 7.1

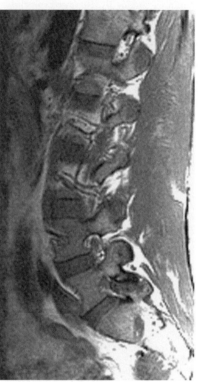

FIGURE 7.2

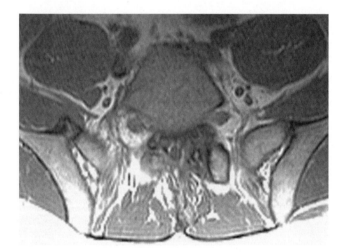

FIGURE 7.3

HISTORY

A 42-year-old with low back and left leg pain.

FINDINGS

Sagittal T1-weighted image on the right (Fig. 7.1) shows diminished size of the right facet joint, at the L5–S1 level (*arrow*). The remainder of the facets are normal in size and morphology. Parasagittal T1-weighted image from the left (Fig. 7.2) shows enlargement of the left facet joint with concomitant foraminal stenosis due to incursion by the superior articular facet from S1. Axial T1-weighted image (Fig. 7.3) confirms the small size of the right facet and the enlargement of the left facet with foraminal stenosis.

DIAGNOSIS

Unilateral hypoplastic facet with compensatory contralateral hypertrophy.

DISCUSSION

Congenital variations in the posterior elements are not infrequent and can take a variety of forms. The most common minor congenital variation is the orientation of the facet joints, which may vary from side to side at the same level. This is called *facet tropism*. The next most common congenital variation is the number of mobile lumbar segments, the so-called transitional lumbosacral body. This may be either lumbarization of S1, giving six lumbar-type bodies, or sacralization of L5, giving four lumbar-type bodies. There may also be partial sacralization of one side. The partial or hemisacralization has been implicated in back pain, thought secondary to increased stress at L4–5 (Bertolotti's syndrome). Congenital hypoplasia or complete absence of a facet may occur, with resultant abnormal increased stresses on the opposite facet. That scenario has occurred in this case, with a hypoplastic right facet giving rise to a compensatory hypertropic left facet. The accelerated degenerative change on the left has led to foraminal bony stenosis.

BIBLIOGRAPHY

Grenier N, Kressel HY, Schiebler ML, et al. Normal and degenerative posterior spinal structures: MR imaging. *Radiology* 1987;165:517–525.
Liang MH, Katz JN, Frymoyer JW. Plain radiographs in evaluating the spine. In: Frymoyer JW, ed. *The adult spine: principles and practice.* New York: Raven Press, 1991.

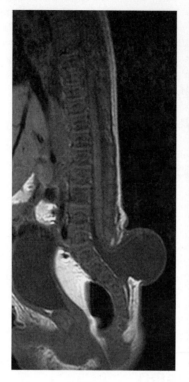 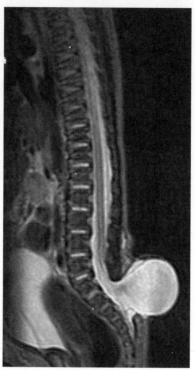

FIGURE 8.1 FIGURE 8.2

HISTORY

A newborn with abnormal prenatal ultrasound.

FINDINGS

Sagittal T1-weighted image (Fig. 8.1) and sagittal T2-weighted images (Fig. 8.2) show a well-defined mass demonstrating CSF signal intensity arising from the posterior aspect of the caudal thecal sac overlying the lumbosacral junction. Nerve roots are seen extending along the posterior margin of the thecal sac and dorsally into the fluid-filled structure. The rest of the vertebral bodies are normal. The conus is low in position but without syrinx or other intradural mass.

DIAGNOSIS

Myelomeningocele.

DISCUSSION

Myelomeningocele is the most common form of spinal dysraphism, characterized by overexpansion of the subarachnoid space with herniation of neural tissue through a large, bony defect dorsally. The cord is tethered at the defect or site of other structural anomalies. This is thought to be secondary to lack of closure at the posterior neuropore at approximately 3 weeks of gestation. Instead of a hollow tube forming during neurolation, the neuro plate remains with a ventral and dorsal surface, the configuration that is called a *neural placode*. The ventral and dorsal roots exit ventrally, since the spinal cord is splayed open. Myelomeningoceles occur at a rate of one per 1000 live births and are slightly more common in girls than in boys. Clinically, the patients have weakness and paralysis of lower extremities and neurogenic bladder. Myelomeningocele is invariably associated with a Chiari II malformation in 99% of cases. This can result in hydrocephalus requiring shunting. Other anomalies include syringohydromyelia and duplication of the central canal. Diastematomyelia has also been associated with this. Follow-up MRs tend to be obtained in children who have had closure of their defect but who exhibit a progressive neurologic deficit. Worsening of bowel or bladder function and loss of previous staple sensory or motor function may be clues. The primary diagnosis requires looking for the site of tethering, as well as any associated intradural masses.

BIBLIOGRAPHY

Byrd SE, Darling CF, McLone DG. Developmental disorders of the pediatric spine. *Radiol Clin North Am* 1991;29:711–752.

Goske MJ, Modic MT, Yu S. Pediatric spine: normal anatomy and spinal dysraphism. In: Modic MT, Masaryk TJ, Ross JS, eds. *Magnetic resonance imaging of the spine*. St Louis: Mosby-Year Book, 1998.

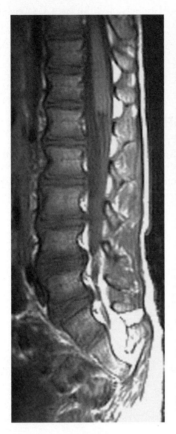 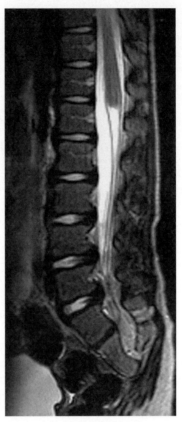

FIGURE 9.1   FIGURE 9.2

HISTORY

A 10-year-old with urinary retention.

FINDINGS

Sagittal T1-weighted (Fig. 9.1) and sagittal T2-weighted (Fig. 9.2) images show truncation of the caudal aspect of the conus, which has a flat or triangular-shaped inferior margin. The roots of the cauda equina have extended inferiorly from this blunted conus. Vertebral bodies below the S2 level are absent. Vertebral bodies, intravertebral disk, and posterior elements above that are relatively normal.

DIAGNOSIS

Caudal regression.

DISCUSSION

Caudal regression syndrome is a group of anomalies affecting the hind end of the trunk, including agenesis of all or portions of the thoracolumbosacral spine, imperforate anus, malformed genitalia, bilateral renal aplasia or dysplasia, pulmonary hypoplasia, and hydromyelia. The spinal involvement ranges from isolated asymptomatic coccygeal aplasia to absent sacral, lumbar, and thoracic vertebrae with severe neurologic deficits. Patients with more extensive vertebral regression will have more severe associated abnormalities. The most common type consists of partial bilaterally segmentric sacral agenesis. The caudal regression syndrome occurs in one of 7500 births. In general, regression above the T10 level is incompatible with life. The syndrome is seen in 1% of offspring of diabetic mothers. However, 16% of patients with caudal regression are offspring of diabetic mothers.

Patients frequently present with orthopedic problems (hip dislocations and equinovarus deformities of the feet) and urinary symptoms secondary to impairment of detrusor function (seen with absence of more than one sacral segment and urologic anomalies). Neurologic manifestations include motor and sensory deficits that usually correspond to the level of vertebral agenesis. Progressive neurologic symptoms may result from dural sac stenosis, narrowed caudal-most bony canal, cord compression by vertebral bony excrescences, lipomyelomeningocele or myelomeningocele, tight filum syndrome, lipoma, diastematomyelia, and adhesive arachnoid bands. Many of these entities may be amenable to surgical correction. Static neurologic symptoms may result from cord or nerve root dysplasias.

Both CT and plain films depict well the associated bony abnormalities, such as hemivertebrae, hypoplastic vertebrae, and unsegmented bars. They can also accurately determine the level of vertebral agenesis and show associated spinal stenosis immediately above the level of agenesis. Magnetic resonance imaging can be used to evaluate these patients and determine the level of termination agenesis. The distal-most cord segment has an abrupt end without tapering. Barkovich et al. initially described this "wedge-shaped cord terminus" in six of 17 patients with caudal regression. The terminal cord is blunted and is longer dorsally than ventrally, distinctly dissimilar to the normal gradual tapered conus.

BIBLIOGRAPHY

Barkovich AJ, Raghavan N, Chuang S, et al. The wedge-shaped cord terminus: a radiographic sign of caudal regression. *Am J Neuroradiol* 1989;10:1223–1231.

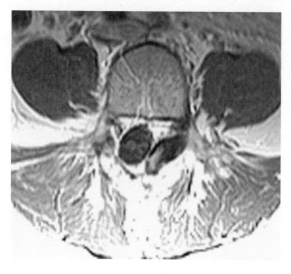

FIGURE 10.1

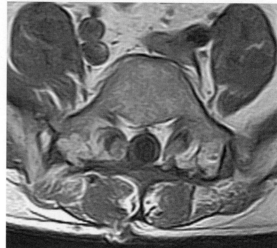

FIGURE 10.2

HISTORY

Two patients with failed back surgery syndrome, with continued back/leg pain.

FINDINGS

In the first of two patients the axial T1-weighted image at the L3 level (Fig. 10.1) shows abnormal central clumping of the roots of the cauda equina. The patient has had a laminectomy, as evidenced by a lack of dorsal elements. In the second patient the axial T1-weighted image (Fig. 10.2) also shows a laminectomy defect at the L5–S1 levels. There is abnormal clumping of the roots along the periphery of the dura with the central portion of the thecal sac showing homogeneous CSF signal intensity.

DIAGNOSIS

Arachnoiditis.

DISCUSSION

MR can identify the varied patterns of lumbar arachnoiditis. These may be classified into three categories or patterns, although this is a spectrum, and patterns may overlap. The first pattern is central adhesion of the nerve roots within the thecal sac into a central clump of soft tissue. Instead of demonstrating their normal feathery pattern, the nerve roots are clumped into one or more cords. The second pattern is adhesion of the nerve roots to the meninges, giving rise to an "empty thecal sac" sign. On MR, only the homogeneous signal of the CSF is present within the thecal sac, and the nerve roots are peripherally attached to the meninges. In the third pattern, as an end stage of the in-

flammatory response, the arachnoiditis becomes an inflammatory mass that fills the thecal sac. On myelography, this type of arachnoiditis is a block, with an irregular "candle-dripping" appearance.

Differential problems involving arachnoiditis include the following:

1. Distinguishing the inflammatory mass from intradural neoplasm. The two can look identical on MR. The separating points are the history and the tendency of arachnoiditis not to enhance with Gd-DTPA to the degree that tumor does.

2. Distinguishing CSF tumor spread from the central clumping pattern. Arachnoiditis tends to be smooth and fairly symmetric in appearance. Drop metastases are more irregular in pattern and enhance to a much greater degree than arachnoiditis.
3. Distinguishing stenosis from arachnoiditis. Bony canal stenosis may give a pattern similar to central clumping from arachnoiditis. However, the obvious extradural degenerative disease causing the compression is easily defined by MR. Superimposed arachnoiditis in these patients cannot be excluded.

BIBLIOGRAPHY

Bangert BA, Ross JS. Arachnoiditis affecting the lumbosacral spine. *Neuroimaging Clin North Am* 1993;3:517–524.

Benoist M, Ficat C, Baraf P, et al. Postoperative lumbar epiduro-arachnoiditis: diagnostic and therapeutic aspects. *Spine* 1980;5:432–436.

Matsui H, Tsuji H, Kanamori M, et al. Laminectomy-induced arachnoradiculitis: a postoperative serial MRI study. *Neuroradiology* 1995;37:660–666.

Ross JS, Masaryk TJ, Modic MT, et al. MR imaging of lumbar arachnoiditis. *Am J Roentgenol* 1987;149:1025–1032.

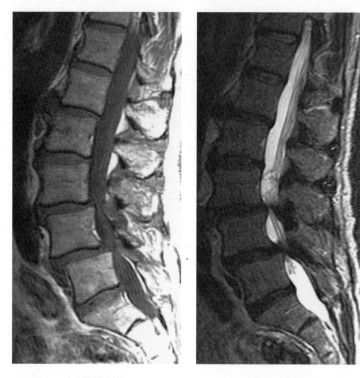

FIGURE 11.1   FIGURE 11.2

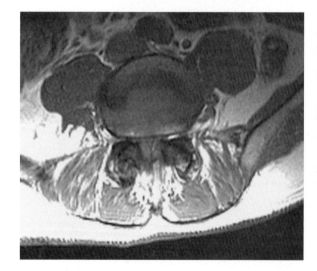

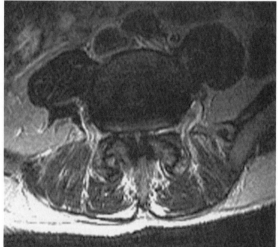

FIGURE 11.3   FIGURE 11.4

HISTORY

A 77-year-old being evaluated for claudication.

FINDINGS

Sagittal T1-weighted (Fig. 11.1) and sagittal T2-weighted (Fig. 11.2) images of the lumbar spine show marked narrowing of the thecal sac at the L3–4 and L4–5 levels. This is confirmed on the axial T1-weighted (Fig.

11.3) and axial T2-weighted fast spin echo (Fig. 11.4) images. The central stenosis is due to diffuse bulging of the anulus fibrosis at both levels, coupled with marked facet and ligamentous hypertrophic change posterior laterally. The ligaments are well demonstrated on the axial fast spin echo sequence as low signal intensity along the posterior lateral margins of the thecal sac. The thecal sac is very small and trefoil in appearance. There is tortuosity to the intrathecal nerve roots; this is particularly noticeable in the sagittal fast spin echo T2-weighted image above the L3–4 level. There is also degenerative spondylolisthesis of L3 on L4 and L4 on L5.

DIAGNOSIS

Lumbar canal stenosis.

DISCUSSION

Spinal stenosis refers to narrowing of the central spinal canal, neural foramina, or lateral recesses. Most commonly, it is acquired secondary to degenerative disease of the intervertebral disk and/or facets, although occasionally developmentally shortened pedicles are an important component of symptomatic spinal stenosis in patients with otherwise mild degenerative changes. The clinical features of spinal stenosis are varied. Most commonly, patients with central canal stenosis present with low back pain, neurogenic claudication, and bilateral sciatica that is often relieved by bending forward. Prior to the development of MR imaging, plain films and CT were used to diagnose spinal stenosis by measuring the dimensions of the bony canal. Currently, the use of such measurements is not recommended. These measurements do not take into account the normal anatomic variation between patients or the role of the disk and ligamentum flava in spinal stenosis, and as such are inaccurate predictors of clinical symptoms. MR imaging accurately depicts the degree and cause of thecal sac narrowing in patients with central canal stenosis. Such narrowing is most commonly due to bony and ligamentous hypertrophy. More severe degrees of narrowing cause central grouping of the nerve roots and dampened CSF pulsations within the thecal sac, both of which can contribute to a confusing pattern of mild increased CSF signal on T1-weighted images. This should not be confused with the presence of arachnoiditis or an intradural mass. Developmental canal narrowing in congenital disorders such as achondroplasia and Morquio's syndrome, and spondylolisthesis, trauma, and Paget's disease are other, less common causes of spinal stenosis.

In addition to central canal stenosis, stenosis of the lateral recess is an important cause of lower-extremity pain and paresthesias. The lateral recess is bordered anteriorly by the posterior aspect of the vertebral body and disc, laterally by the pedicle, and posteriorly by the superior articular facet. The root sleeve within the lateral recess is often compressed by bony hypertrophy of the superior facet, often in combination with disk bulging and osteophyte along the anterior border of the lateral recess. Lateral recess disease can clinically mimic disk herniation. MR imaging allows differentiation between central and lateral recess stenosis and provides important information for presurgical planning.

BIBLIOGRAPHY

Airaksinen O, Herno A, Turunen V, et al. Surgical outcome of 438 patients treated surgically for lumbar spinal stenosis. *Spine* 1997;22:2278–2282.

Amunosen T, Weber H, Lilleas F, et al. Lumbar spinal stenosis: clinical and radiologic features. *Spine* 1995;20:1178–1186.

Borenstein DG. Epidemiology, etiology, diagnostic evaluation, and treatment of low back pain. *Curr Opin Rheumatol* 1997;9:144–150.

Porter RW. Spinal stenosis and neurogenic claudication. *Spine* 1996;21:2046–2052.

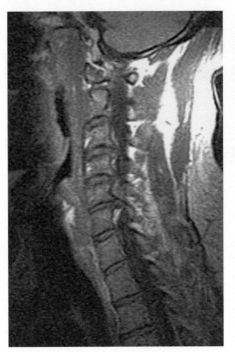

FIGURE 12.1

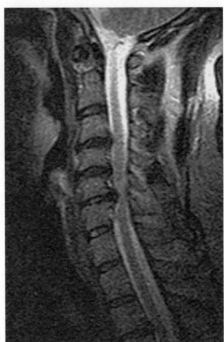

FIGURE 12.2

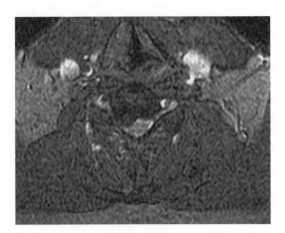

FIGURE 12.3

HISTORY

A 35-year-old with right arm pain.

FINDINGS

These sagittal T1-weighted (Fig. 12.1), sagittal T2-weighted (Fig. 12.2), and axial two-dimensional gradient echo (Fig. 12.3) images were obtained from a low-field (0.2 Tesla) system. There is a relatively isointense lesion at the C5–6 level on the right on the T1-weighted images showing a low signal on the T2 and gradient echo images. This effaces the right anterolateral aspect of the thecal sac and extends into the right neural foramen. Smaller disk protrusion is seen at the C3–4 level with mild effacement of the sac but no evidence of cord compromise.

DIAGNOSIS

Cervical disk herniation.

DISCUSSION

MR has made a tremendous impact in the evaluation of cervical degenerative disk disease because of the high contrast between foraminal or epidural fat and disk material or osteophyte coupled with its multiplanar imaging capability. The intrinsic contrast and good spatial resolution permit accurate assessment of herniations and stenosis, with MR correctly predicting surgical findings in 74% of patients, whereas CT myelography was correct in 85% and plain-film myelography in 67% (Modic et al). In a blinded retrospective review, Brown et al. studied 34 patients with MR who underwent operation. In the cervical spine, MR correctly predicted 88% of the surgically proven lesions in comparison with 81% for postmyelographic CT, 58% for myelography, and 50% for CT. Small osteophytes were sometimes not predicted on MR, although these were visible on plain films. MR replaced the invasive myelographic evaluation in 32% of the operated patients. The MR technique included T1-weighted images in both the sagittal and axial planes with a 5-mm slice thickness and intersection gap of 1 mm. Sagittal T2-weighted images were obtained only in selected patients. Brown et al. concluded that MRI combined with plain films provides an accurate and noninvasive test for cervical radiculopathy and myelopathy.

Imaging protocols for MR of cervical degenerative disease tend to vary widely from institution to institution with regard to specific imaging parameters. However, there are common themes based on the need for contrast between disk and cerebrospinal fluid (CSF), the need for several imaging planes, and time constraints. Usually, protocols provide for a T1-weighted two-dimensional spin echo sagittal image, which provides detailed gross anatomy with dark CSF and high signal intensity marrow. Then two-dimensional axial and sagittal images with high-signal-intensity CSF (the "CSF myelogram" effect) are often acquired that highlight any anterior extradural disease and its effect on the thecal sac. This type of image contrast can be obtained with either spin echo T2 or gradient echo T2* imaging.

BIBLIOGRAPHY

Brant ZM, Jensen MC, Obuchowski N, et al. Interobserver and intraobserver variability in interpretation of lumbar disc abnormalities: a comparison of two nomenclatures. *Spine* 1995;20:1257–1264.

Brown BM, Schwartz RH, Frank E, et al. Preoperative evaluation of cervical radiculopathy and myelopathy by surface-coil MR imaging. *Am J Neuroradiol* 1988;9:859–866.

Modic MT, Masaryk TJ, Mulopulos GP, et al. Cervical radiculopathy: CT with metrizamide and metrizamide myelography. *Radiology* 1986;161:573–579.

Modic MT, Masaryk TJ, Ross JS, et al. Imaging of degenerative disk disease. *Radiology* 1988;168:177–186.

Modic MT, Ross JS, Masaryk TJ. Imaging of degenerative disease of the cervical spine. *Clin Orthop* 1989;239:109–120.

Modic MT, Ross JS, Obuchowski NA, et al. Contrast-enhanced MR imaging in acute lumbar radiculopathy: a pilot study of the natural history. *Radiology* 1995;195:429–435.

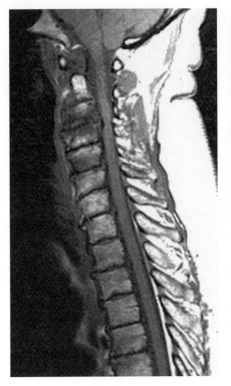

FIGURE 13.1

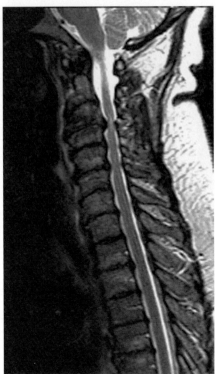

FIGURE 13.2

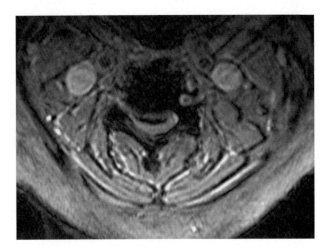

FIGURE 13.3

HISTORY

A 69-year-old with myelopathy.

FINDINGS

Sagittal T1-weighted image (Fig. 13.1) shows diffuse degenerative disease with loss of disk space height at multiple levels. This appears particularly severe at the C3–4 level and is confirmed on the sagittal fast spin echo T2-weighted image (Fig. 13.2). The axial gradient echo 3D sequence (Fig. 13.3) confirms a severe central canal stenosis due principally to osteophyte with marked narrowing of the thecal sac. The sagittal fast spin echo T2-weighted image shows high signal within the cervical cord at the C3–4 level.

DIAGNOSIS

Cervical spondylosis with focal myelomalacia.

DISCUSSION

Cervical spondylotic myelopathy is the most common cause of cord dysfunction in patients over 50 years of age. The first large series was reported in 1952 by Brain et al. Cervical spondylotic myelopathy is part of the spectrum of degenerative changes occurring in the cervical spine, including pain, radiculopathy, and myelopathy. The physical examination of cervical spondylotic myelopathy includes both upper and lower motor neuron signs. Lower motor neuron signs occur at the level of the lesion and produce weakness and hyporeflexia in the upper extremities. Upper motor neuron signs are seen below the lesion level, since the long tracks are involved. This produces spasticity and hyperreflexia in the lower extremities. Additionally, sensory findings can be found due to compression of the spinothalamic tracks, posterior columns, or dorsal nerve roots.

Several clinical syndromes are involved in cervical spondylotic myelopathy. These include (a) The lateral or radicular syndrome, where nerve root symptoms predominate; (b) the medial or myelopathic syndrome, which involves long tract signs; (c) the combined syndrome, involving both radicular and myelopathic signs (the most common presentation); (d) the vascular syndrome, related to the variable injury within the cord due to ischemia; and (e) the anterior syndrome, which produces painless weakness in the upper extremities. Myelopathy can also be classified based upon the spinal cord tracts that are involved. This classification may be divided into five types:

1. The most common is the transverse lesion that involves the posterior columns, spinothalamic, and corticospinal tracts.
2. The motor system is involved, including the corticospinal tracts. This produces upper- and lower-extremity weakness and spasticity.
3. The central cord syndrome, which classically is described as producing upper-extremity weakness that is greater than the lower-extremity weakness. The hand weakness tends to be profound.
4. The Brown-Sequard syndrome, which is due to unilateral compression of the cord and produces ipsilateral hemiparesis and contralateral pain and temperature loss.
5. The brachialgia cord syndrome, which produces upper-extremity root compression with long tract findings due to cord compression.

MEASUREMENTS

Various measurements have been applied to evaluating cervical spondylotic myelopathy. While it is tempting to try to put a strict number on this disease, its application in any one person tends to be quite problematic. Various studies have shown that the canal is reduced in patients with cervical spondylotic myelopathy. The normal diameter of the canal from C3 to C7 is approximately 17 mm and is decreased to 13 mm in cervical spondylotic myelopathy. However, the range of size associated with myelopathy has varied from 10 mm up to 14 mm. The ratio of the AP canal diameter to the vertebral body diameter has been used to assess myelopathy. This "Pavlov ratio" (sometimes referred to as the *Torg ratio*) is normal if it is 1.0 or greater. A ratio of 0.8 or less is considered abnormal. Additionally, myelopathic symptoms tend to occur when the canal cross-sectional area is less than 60 mm. Cervical spondylotic myelopathy has a chronic progressive course. In general, no patients return to the normal state once the progression of symptomatology occurs. Seventy-five percent of patients have episodic worsening, with a steplike degenerative process in between quiescent periods that can be of either long or short duration. Approximately 24% of patients show a slow, steady progression of their symptomatology, with 5% having a rapid onset. There does not appear to be any relationship between the age of onset and the overall prognosis.

BIBLIOGRAPHY

Brain WR, Northfield D, Wilkinson M. The neurological manifestations of cervical spondylosis. *Brain* 1952;75:187–225.

Crandall PH, Batzdorf U. Cervical spondylotic myelopathy. J Neurosurg 1966;25:57.

Masaryk TJ, Modic MT, Geisinger MA, et al. Cervical myelopathy: a comparison of magnetic resonance and myelography. *J Comput Assist Tomogr* 1986;10:184–194.

Modic MT, Ross JS, Masaryk TJ. Imaging of degenerative disease of the cervical spine. *Clin Orthop* 1989;239:109–120.

Pavlov H, Torg JS, Robie B, et al. Cervical spinal stenosis: determination with vertebral body ratio method. *Radiology* 1987;164:771–775.

Ross JS. Myelopathy. *Neuroimaging Clin North Am* 1995;5:367–384.

Statham PF, Hadley DM, Macpherson P, et al. MRI in the management of suspected cervical spondylotic myelopathy. *J Neurol Neurosurg Psychiatry* 1991;54:484–489.

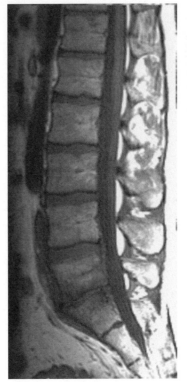 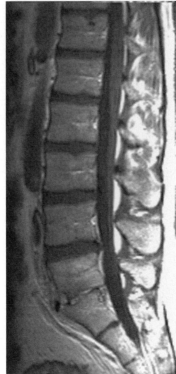 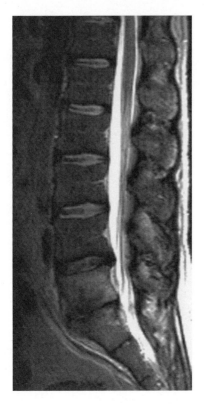

| FIGURE 14.1 | FIGURE 14.2 | FIGURE 14.3 |

HISTORY

A 47-year-old with back pain.

FINDINGS

Sagittal T1-weighted image without contrast (Fig. 14.1) shows a marked loss of disk space height at L5–S1. End plates appear maintained and seen as low signal intensity. Sagittal T1-weighted image following contrast administration (Fig. 14.2) shows fairly heterogeneous enhancement within the intervertebral disk itself, including a Schmorl's node along the anterior inferior end plate at L5. Sagittal fast spin echo T2-weighted image (Fig. 14.3) shows mild increase signal within the L5 and S1 bodies with very little high signal within the intervertebral disk itself. There is also a small protrusion of the intervertebral disk at L4–5 with mild effacement of the thecal sac.

DIAGNOSIS

Degenerative end-plate change mimics disk space infection.

DISCUSSION

A couple of dilemmas can occur in the diagnosis of disk space infection with MR and are related to the changes that may occur in the vertebral bodies and end plates in association with disk degeneration. The first problem that can occur is the potential "masking" of the usual low-signal-intensity changes of disk space infection on T1-weighted MR images by superimposed high-signal-intensity type II degenerative end-plate changes. Correlation with the T2-weighted images would help make the diagnosis in this scenario, showing abnormal increased signal intensity within the disk space with disk space infection. Second, type I end-plate changes associated with degeneration have similar signal changes involving the vertebral bodies, as do disk space infection. The differential point in this case is the usual low-signal disk space seen with degeneration on T2-weighted images, as opposed to the high-signal-intensity disk seen with infection. However, this is not foolproof, and problems occur when the type I end-plate changes are associated with a degenerated disk that contains cystic areas, which are increased in signal on T2-weighted images. Enhancement can occur within the disk with both disk space infection and degenerative disease. In these cases, differentiation from early disk space infection might be impossible.

BIBLIOGRAPHY

Modic MT, Steinberg PM, Ross JS, et al. Degenerative disk disease: assessment of changes in vertebral body marrow with MR imaging. *Radiology* 1988;166:193–199.

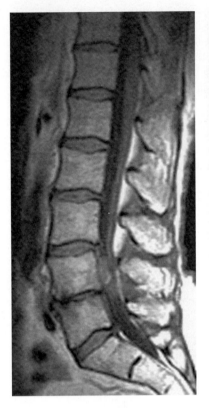

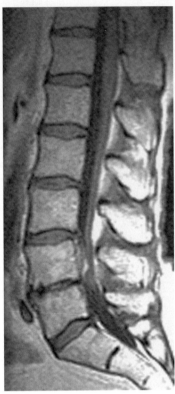

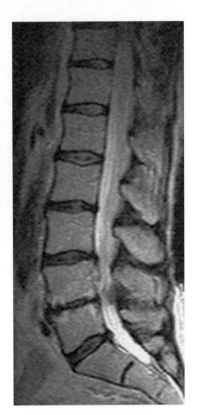

FIGURE 15.1

FIGURE 15.2

FIGURE 15.3

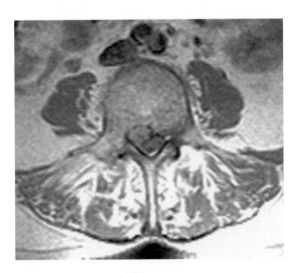

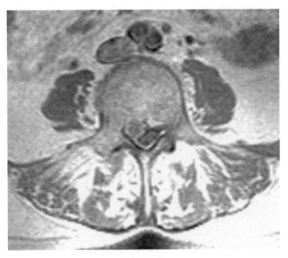

FIGURE 15.4

FIGURE 15.5

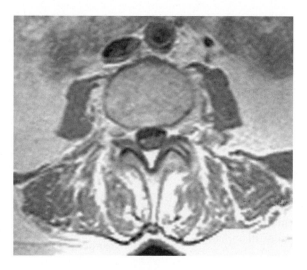

FIGURE 15.6

HISTORY

A 50-year-old with right leg pain.

FINDINGS

Sagittal T1-weighted image without contrast (Fig. 15.1) shows a large isointense (to disk) mass at the L4 level posterior to the vertebral body. This appears contiguous with the inferior margin of the L3–4 intervertebral disk. The lesion appears extradural and effaces the cauda equina at the L4 level. Following contrast administration, the sagittal T1-weighted image (Fig. 15.2) shows mild peripheral enhancement surrounding the soft-tissue lesion at L4. The fast spin echo T2-weighted image (Fig. 15.3) shows the lesion to extend inferiorly from the L3–4 disk level and shows slightly diminished signal intensity. Axial T1-weighted image before contrast (Fig. 15.4) and after contrast (Fig. 15.5) shows peripheral enhancement surrounding the right anterior epidural lesion. There is effacement of the right lateral aspect of the thecal sac. Higher up, at the L3 body level (Fig. 15.6), there is enhancement of a solitary intradural nerve.

DIAGNOSIS

Lumbar herniation with enhancing intradural nerve.

DISCUSSION

Jinkins et al. first identified MR enhancement of intradural nerve roots with gadolinium-based contrast material. He looked at 200 consecutive patients with 0.1 mmol/kg of contrast material. In 5% of cases, there were enhancing nerve roots, but 21.2% enhancement when there was a focal disk protrusion. He put forth the theory that MR with contrast allows direct visualization of the disruption of the blood nerve barrier, which could be associated with pain and clinical symptomatology. There was generally good correlation with symptoms and site of root enhancement. Other studies have added to the interest in root enhancement. Crisi et al. evaluated 20 patients with herniated disks and found ipsilateral root enhancement in 30%. They noted that a pattern of strong ipsilateral root enhancement was different from the diffuse minimal enhancement found in normal intrathecal roots (which was seen in 55% of their patients). They considered this a transient phenomenon of the acute phase of herniation. Toyone evaluated 25 patients with sciatica and found 25 herniations (0.1 mmol/kg at 0.5 Tesla). In this study, 17 of 25 patients showed root enhancement. They also saw a trend of increased root enhancement with a positive straight leg raise of less than 30 degrees, versus less root enhancement with an increased straight leg raise angle. The hope upon seeing this root enhancement is that it would indicate active disruption and active radiculitis. This radiculitis might correlate with the side and site of compression and may reflect sites active radiculopathy and of "pain production."

However, several factors conspire to muddy the initially clean premise of the potential utility of this finding of root enhancement. Current problems with the theory regarding implementation of this finding in any one patient include the following:

1. Jinkins et al. noted that of the seven patients with disk-protrusive disease, four had ipsilateral pathology to the clinical findings but three showed either midline disease, contralateral disease, or bulging disk. Additionally, single-root radiculopathy can show multiple-root enhancement and multiple-root enhancement could be caused by many etiologies, such as low-grade inflammation, autoimmune, and toxic factors.

2. Crisi et al. could not find a clinical correlate to the enhancement, with a wide overlap of pain with or without the presence of root enhancement. They concluded that whether the blood nerve barrier of compressed roots breaks down was of little importance, with no immediate clinical utility to the finding.

3. Nerve root enhancement reflects enhancement of vessels and is not related, or only indirectly related, to intrinsic nerve pathology. Lane and Koeller scanned 30 asymptomatic volunteers and showed that 63% had lumbar nerve root enhancement. In 95% of the cases, there was associated flow-related enhancement that was eliminated with superiorly situated saturation pulse (proving that it relates to flow within a macroscopic vessel, and not solid tissue). They concluded that this represents intravascular enhancement of caudally draining radicular veins and that caution was needed in ascribing enhancement directly to intrinsic root disease.

4. An additional confounding item is the change in visibility of root enhancement with increasing contrast dosage. Jinkins et al. presented their experience with 0.3 mmol/kg of contrast in the lumbar spine. This study found that 10 of 11 subjects showed "normal" enhancement of the lumbosacral nerve roots. They concluded that this dosage was too large for evaluation of suspected pathology involving the nerve roots and leptomeninges. Crisi et al. also reported on normal root enhancement in their population using only 0.1 mmol/kg of contrast material. Obviously, many factors may be involved in calling a nerve root enhancing, such as magnet field strength, specific sequence used (vanilla spin echo imaging versus magnetization transfer contrast), and intravenous contrast dosage.

As with all incomplete knowledge, more questions are raised by these studies than can currently be answered. Some "root" enhancement is undoubtedly related to vessels, such as the radicular veins. Also undoubtedly, enhancement of the "root" is correlated with disk compressive disease. Whether this enhancement is related to vascular congestion, stasis, or intrinsic blood nerve barrier disruption (or both) is unknown.

BIBLIOGRAPHY

Crisi G, Carpeggiani P, Trevisan C. Gadolinium-enhanced nerve roots in lumbar disk herniation. *Am J Neuroradiol* 1993;14:1379–1392.

Jinkins JR, Osborn AG, Garrett D, et al. Spinal nerve enhancement with Gd-DTPA: MR correlation with the postoperative lumbosacral spine. *Am J Neuroradiol* 1993;14:383–394.

Lane JI, Koeller KK, Atkinson JL. Contrast-enhanced radicular veins on MR of the lumbar spine in an asymptomatic study group. *Am J Neuroradiol* 1995;16:269–273.

Toyone T, Takahashi K, Kitahara H, et al. Visualisation of symptomatic nerve roots: prospective study of contrast-enhanced MRI in patients with lumbar disc herniation. *J Bone Joint Surg Br* 1993;75:529–533.

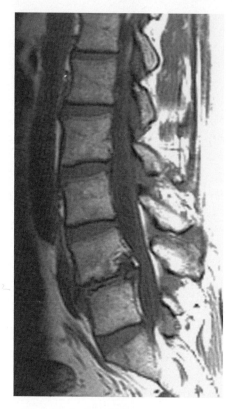

FIGURE 16.1

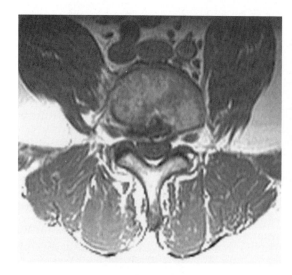

FIGURE 16.2

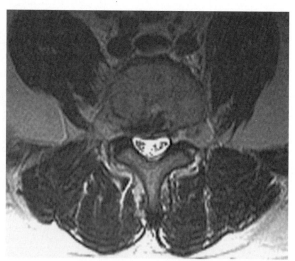

FIGURE 16.3

<u>HISTORY</u>

A 26-year-old with back/leg pain.

FINDINGS

Sagittal T1 (Fig. 16.1) and axial T1 (Fig. 16.2) images of the lumbar spine demonstrate a focal linear of high signal intensity along the posterior inferior aspect of the L4 body extending into the anterior epidural space. A linear area of low signal separates this fragment from the remainder of the L4 body. Disk material extending along with this fragment at the L4–5 level is seen as low signal intensity on the axial T2-weighted fast spin echo image (Fig. 16.3). There is also degeneration of the L4–5 disk with loss of disk space height and evidence of the vacuum phenomenon or calcification.

DIAGNOSIS

Type II limbus fracture with herniation.

DISCUSSION

A limbus vertebral body is defined as having a defect in the margins of the body with a detached triangular bony fragment. This occurs at the margins of the superior or inferior vertebral end plates. Most of these types of fractures are attributed to disk material herniating into the vertebral body or the cartilaginous end plate at the bony rim. Fragmentation of the body can occur and can be associated with a disk herniation. The anterior superior margin of midlumbar vertebral bodies is most commonly affected. These have been classified into three types. Type I is a posterior cortical avulsion, where there is a separation of the entire margin that is seen as a calcific arc on CT with no evidence of associated large bony fracture. In type II there is an avulsion fracture of a portion of the vertebral body substance, including the margin (cortical and cancellous), which may have annular rim and cartilage. Type III fractures are more laterally localized and include smaller posterior irregularities of the end plate. These types of fractures are classically found in adolescents and young adults. This occurs since ossification at the site of the vertebral ring apophysis and the cartilaginous rim is incomplete until the age of 18 to 25. Epstein et al. introduced a type IV lesion, where the fracture spans the entire length of the vertebral body along its posterior margin and is not confined at the superior or inferior margin of the disk space. Trauma may play a role, with injuries occurring during weightlifting or gymnastics and as a result of motor vehicle accidents. Other cases show no definite insighting event. Patients with these types of fractures often have a large amount of back and leg pain and muscle spasm, with relatively few neurologic findings. The L4–5 level is the typical location. The key imaging finding is the fact of the fracture fragment associated with the herniation; that is, that this is not a simple herniation, because a portion of the thecal sac compromise is due to bone. Separating a routine disk herniation from a limbus fracture can be very difficult, with MR failing to define this abnormality in 38 instances out of 49 in the series reported by Epstein in 1992.

BIBLIOGRAPHY

Epstein NE. Lumbar surgery for 56 limbus fractures emphasizing noncalcified type III lesions. *Spine* 1992;17:1489–1496.

Epstein NE. Treatment of fractures of the vertebral limbus and spinal stenosis in 5 adolescents and 5 adults. *Neurosurgery* 1989;24:595–604.

Takata K. Fracture of the posterior margin of a lumbar vertebral body. *J Bone Joint Surg Am* 1988;70:589–594.

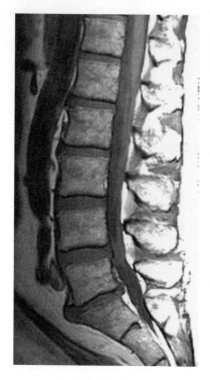

FIGURE 17.1

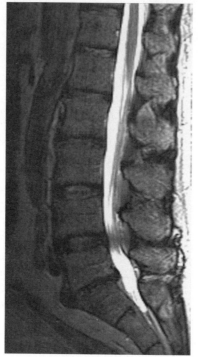

FIGURE 17.2

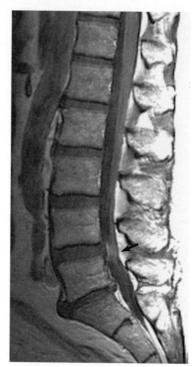

FIGURE 17.3

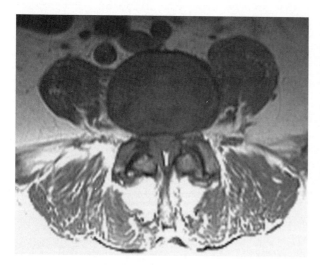

FIGURE 17.4

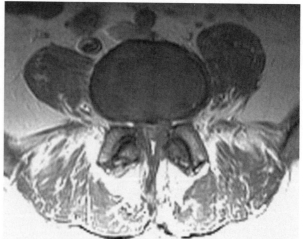

FIGURE 17.5

HISTORY

A 40-year-old with bilateral leg pain/numbness.

FINDINGS

Sagittal T1-weighted (Fig. 17.1) and sagittal fast spin echo T2-weighted (Fig. 17.2) images show ill-defined soft-tissue signal within the region of the thecal sac at the L4–5 level. There is a broad-base disk bulge at L5–S1. Following contrast administration (Fig. 17.3), there is enhancement that appears intradural at the L4–5 level (*arrow*). Axial T1-weighted image prior to contrast (Fig. 17.4) shows severe narrowing of the thecal sac into a trefoil pattern, resulting from the diffuse bulging of the annulus anteriorly and facet and ligamentous hypertrophic change posterolaterally. Axial T1-weighted image following contrast (Fig. 17.5) shows scattered intradural enhancement.

DIAGNOSIS

Lumbar canal stenosis with intradural enhancement.

DISCUSSION

Central stenosis can be broadly divided into either acquired or congenital (developmental) stenosis. Often these two types coexist, with narrowing of the spinal canal combined with facet and ligamentous hypertrophic degenerative change, as well as diffuse bulging of the annulus fibrosis producing a trefoil-shaped and narrowed thecal sac. Central stenosis can occur either with or without associated foraminal stenosis. Post mortem studies have shown in severe canal stenosis the presence of nerve redundancy due to chronic stretching and elongation of the roots. This is not uncommonly seen on myelography and MR imaging. Pathology has shown changes within these roots such as demyelination, axon loss, and endoneural fibrosis. Central canal stenosis of the lumbar spine can produce the clinical symptom of neurogenic claudication. This consists of lower-extremity pain that may be associated with numbness or weakness. The findings are often bilateral. The symptoms are exacerbated by standing erect and are relieved by flexion. Jinkins has shown a variety of patterns of intradural enhancement associated with central spinal canal stenosis. The enhancement pattern could be either linear, curvilinear, punctate, or diffuse. The enhancement probably reflects a combination of dilated venous enhancement as well as intraneural enhancement. This intradural enhancement is thought to reflect unequivocal neuropathology associated with stenotic spinal disease when there is clinical claudication of an ambiguous cause. The differential of intradural enhancement of the cauda equina is extensive and includes leptomeningeal disease (including metastases) and granulomatous disease, as well as meningitis. However, this pattern of focal enhancement as seen within this case, at the level of the central stenosis, is typical as a sequela of the degenerative disease. This pattern of enhancement does not imply a more aggressive underlying pathology.

BIBLIOGRAPHY

Airaksinen O, Herno A, Turunen V, et al. Surgical outcome of 438 patients treated surgically for lumbar spinal stenosis. *Spine* 1997;22:2278–2282.

Jinkins JR. Gd-DTPA enhanced MR of the lumbar spinal canal in patients with claudication. *J Comput Assist Tomogr* 1993;17(4):555–562.

Salibi BS. Neurogenic intermittent claudication and stenosis of the lumbar spinal canal. *Surg Neurol* 1976;5:269.

Suzuki K, Takatsu T, Inoue H, et al. Redundant nerve roots of the cauda equina caused by lumbar spinal canal stenosis. *Spine* 1992;17:1337.

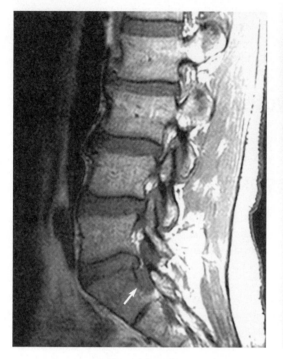

FIGURE 18.1

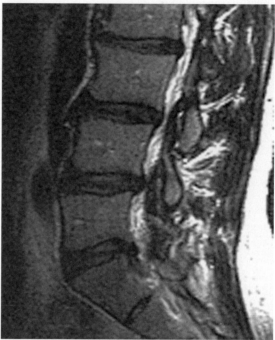

FIGURE 18.2

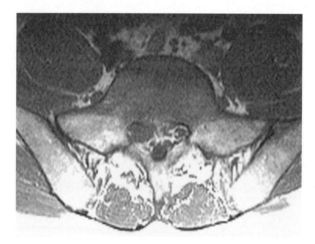

FIGURE 18.3

HISTORY

A 53-year-old with right lower-extremity pain extending below the knee.

FINDINGS

Sagittal T1-weighted (Fig. 18.1) and axial T1-weighted (Fig. 18.3) images show a mass that is isointense to intervertebral disk signal intensity along the exiting course of the right S1 root, seen inferior to the L5–S1 disk space level (*arrow*). This also shows low signal on the T2-weighted sequence (Fig. 18.2) and appears contiguous with the disk space on the T2-weighted image.

DIAGNOSIS

Free disk fragment.

DISCUSSION

Several studies have shown that the size of a disk herniation can reduce dramatically in patients undergoing conservative management. Saal evaluated 11 patients with extrusions and radiculopathy who were all treated nonoperatively. CT studies were obtained in all patients at the inception of treatment and were compared with follow-up MR studies. Eleven percent of patients had a 0 to 50% decrease in size of the herniations, 36% had a 50% to 75% decrease in size, and 46% had a 75% to 100% decrease in size. Maximum shrinkage of extrusion occurred in the cephalocaudal dimension. These authors postulate that with extruded or sequestered disk herniations, reduction in size may be secondary to growth of granulation tissue or alternately due to water imbibition of the extruded nuclear material. Bush et al. evaluated 165 patients presenting with sciatica and were treated with serial epidural administration. CT failed to demonstrate the pathology accounting for symptoms and signs in 4%. Sixty-four of 84 herniated or sequestered disks showed a degree of or complete resolution within 1 year, whereas only seven of 27 bulging disks showed any resolution at 1 year. No correlation was demonstrated between disk resolution and final neurologic outcome. Maigne et al. evaluated 47 patients with acute sciatica undergoing conservative medical therapy consisting of bedrest, steroids, and physical therapy. Five of 47 failed conservative management. Patients were entered into the study after documentation of a positive CT scan. Forty of the patients underwent a second CT scan, 1 to 15 months after the initial episode. Initial CT studies showed 13 small, 20 medium, and 15 large herniations, with the size of the disk being determined with respect to the anterior-posterior dimensions of the lumbar canal. Follow-up studies demonstrated nine of the herniations had decreased by 25%, eight had decreased by 50% to 75%, and 31 had decreased between 75% and 100%. In this study, the large herniations were most likely to decrease in size, and these authors postulate that the larger herniations act as a foreign body in the epidural space and are penetrated by granulation tissue, infiltrated by capillary vessels and transformed into scar. Bozzao et al. evaluated 69 patients with MR-proven lumbar disk herniation that underwent follow-up study. Sixty-three percent of the patients showed a reduction in size of disk herniation (with 48% having reduction of more than 70%), whereas only 8% demonstrated worsening of the clinical picture (which showed an increase in size of disk herniation).

Several papers have described the prevalence of herniated disks in asymptomatic populations. Wiesel et al. evaluated 52 patients with no history of back trouble, mixed randomly with six scans from patients with surgically proven disease utilizing CT. Irrespective of age, 35.4% were found to be "abnormal." Spinal disease was identified in an average 19.5% of those under 40 years of age and was a herniated nucleus pulposus in every instance. In the group of those more than 40 years old, there was an average of 50% "abnormal" findings, with a diagnosis of herniated disk, facet degeneration, and stenosis occurring most frequently. Boden et al. evaluated 67 individuals who had never had low back pain, sciatica, or neurogenic claudication by MRI. Of those patients who were less than 60 years old, 20% had a herniated nucleus pulposus and one had spinal stenosis. In the group of those over 60 years of age, 57% of the scans were abnormal, with 37% of the subjects having a herniated nucleus pulposus and 21% having spinal stenosis. There was degeneration or bulging of a disk at least at one lumbar level in 35% of the subjects between 20 and 39 years of age. Jensen et al. evaluated 98 asymptomatic patients by MRI. Fifty-two percent of such subjects had a bulge at one level at least, 27% had a protrusion, and 1% had an extrusion. All these studies leave unanswered the question of the significance of the morphologic abnormalities and raise the question of the role that disk herniation plays in the symptomatic population.

BIBLIOGRAPHY

Boden SD, Davis DO, Dina TS, et al. Abnormal magnetic resonance scans of the lumbar spine in asymptomatic subjects. *J Bone Joint Surg Am* 1990;72(3):403–408.

Bozzao A, Gallucci M, Masciocchi C, et al. Lumbar disc herniation: MR imaging assessment of natural history in patients treated without surgery. *Radiology* 1992;185:135–141.

Bush K, Cowan N, Katz DE, et al. The natural history of sciatica associated with disc pathology. *Spine* 1992;17:1205–1212.

Jensen M, Brant-Zawadzki M, Obuchowski N, et al. Magnetic resonance imaging of the lumbar spine in people without back pain. *N Engl J Med* 1994;l331:69–73.

Maigne J, Rime B, Delignet B. Computed tomographic follow-up study of forty-eight cases of nonoperatively treated lumbar intervertebral disc herniation. *Spine* 1992;27:1071–1074.

Saal JA, Saal JS, Herzog RJ. The natural history of lumbar intervertebral disc extrusions treated conservatively. *Spine* 1990;15:683–686.

Wiesel SW, Tsourmas N, Feffer HL, et al. A study of computer-assisted tomography. I. The incidence of positive CT scans in an asymptomatic group of patients. 1984 Volvo Award in Clinical Sciences. *Spine* 1984;9:549–551.

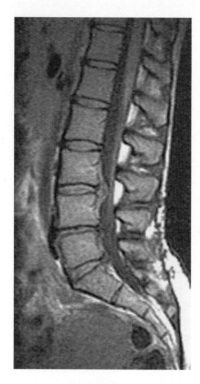

FIGURE 19.1

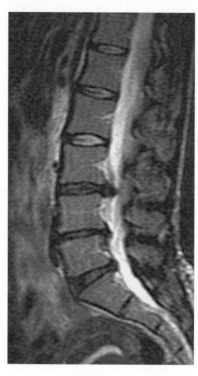

FIGURE 19.2

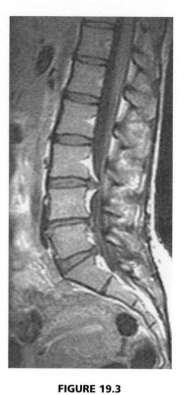

FIGURE 19.3

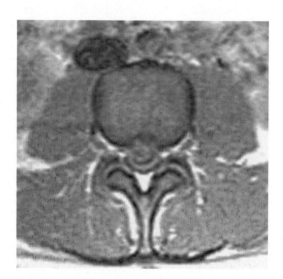

FIGURE 19.4

HISTORY

A 46-year-old with low back pain.

FINDINGS

These images were obtained from a low-field (0.2 Tesla) system. Sagittal T1-weighted image (Fig. 19.1) shows an extradural lesion at the L3–4 level that is contiguous with the disk space. This lesion shows low signal intensity on the T2-weighted sequence (Fig. 19.2) and is getting confirmed to be contiguous with the disk space. Following contrast administration, the sagittal T1-weighted image (Fig. 19.3) shows peripheral enhancement, which extends over the anterior epidural space at the L3–4 levels. These reflect enhancing epidural veins. Axial T1-weighted image without contrast (Fig. 19.4) shows the severe degree of effacement of the thecal sac posteriorly, by the large anterior disk herniation.

DIAGNOSIS

Disk extrusion.

DISCUSSION

In a prospective, blind study in 1986, Modic et al. compared surface-coil MR, CT, and myelography in the evaluation of disk herniation and stenosis. There was an 82.6% agreement between MR and surgical findings for the type and location of the disease. This study also showed an 83% agreement between CT and surgical findings and a 71.8% agreement between myelography and surgery. Canal stenosis, ligamentous hypertrophy, and facet disease can all be demonstrated with MR, with good correlation of the canal size seen by MR with CT. Ross et al. evaluated 30 patients with symptoms suggestive of disk disease; they were evaluated both with and without administration of contrast. Gd-DTPA increased the level of confidence in diagnosis at only one of eight cervical levels and one of 10 lumbar levels; these patients were eventually treated surgically. Although Gd-DTPA's usefulness in the evaluation of lumbar disk disease seems limited, contrast did define enhancement surrounding disk herniations in these patients, who had no previous surgery. Pathology proved these herniations to be associated with granulation or scar tissue. Enhancement surrounding disk herniations would seem to represent a spectrum of the normal reparative process involving granulation tissue. Scar is capable of "digesting" or absorbing disk material and is most intense in the prolapsed portion of the disk. It has been hypothesized that this absorption accounts for the disappearance of symptoms over time. Some pathologists consider vascularization at the edge of disk material to be the only reliable clue that disk prolapse has occurred. It is unknown at present whether this scar tissue regresses or progresses with time and how this relates to the patient's symptomatology and response to treatment, especially conservative management with rest and steroids.

BIBLIOGRAPHY

Brant ZM, Jensen MC, Obuchowski N, et al. Interobserver and intraobserver variability in interpretation of lumbar disc abnormalities: a comparison of two nomenclatures. *Spine* 1995;20:1257–1264.

Modic MT, Masaryk TJ. Lumbar herniated disk disease and canal stenosis: prospective evaluation by surface coil MR, CT, and myelography. *Am J Roentgenol* 1986;147:757.

Ross JS, Modic MT, Masaryk TJ, et al. Assessment of extradural degenerative disease with Gd-DTPA-enhanced MR imaging: correlation with surgical and pathologic findings. *Am J Neuroradiol* 1989;10:1243.

Silverman CS, Lenchik L, Shimkin PM, et al. The value of MR in differentiating subligamentous from supraligamentous lumbar disk herniations. *Am J Neuroradiol* 1995;16:571–579.

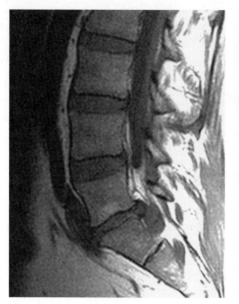

FIGURE 20.1

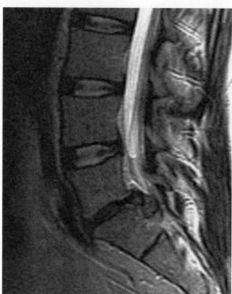

FIGURE 20.2

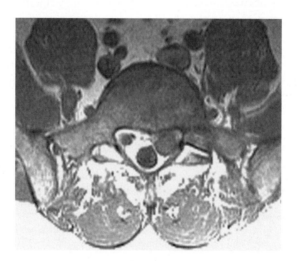

FIGURE 20.3

HISTORY

A 50-year-old with left lancinating lower-extremity pain extending below the knee.

FINDINGS

Sagittal T1-weighted (Fig. 20.1) and sagittal T2-weighted fast spin echo (Fig. 20.2) images show a lobulated soft-tissue lesion adjacent to the L5–S1 intervertebral disk. Axial T1-weighted image (Fig. 20.3) shows the lesion to be well defined and to extend into the region of the exiting left S1 root.

DIAGNOSIS

Free disk fragment.

DISCUSSION

A free fragment, or sequestered disk, is defined as a herniation through a full-thickness defect in the annulus, which is no longer attached to the parent nucleus. This separation is easy to tell at surgery but is much more problematic with MR. Generally, a free fragment is inferred on MR by migration of the disk material away from the parent disk space. Free fragments may lie anterior or posterior to the posterior longitudinal ligament or, rarely, may be intradural. Both ex-truded disks and free fragments may show increased signal intensity on T2-weighted images. Free fragments have definite clinical implications because they (a) can produce misleading clinical signs, (b) are a contraindication to chymopapain injection or percutaneous diskectomy, and (c) may require a more extensive surgical procedure if migration occurs away from the disk space of origin. Intraforaminal and extraforaminal herniations are also well defined by MR.

BIBLIOGRAPHY

Masaryk TJ, Ross JS, Modic MT, et al. High-resolution MR imaging of sequestered lumbar intervertebral disks. *Am J Roentgenol* 1988;150:1155–1162.

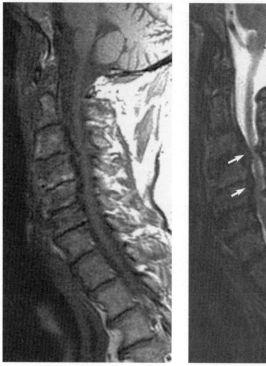

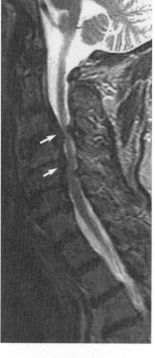

FIGURE 21.1

FIGURE 21.2

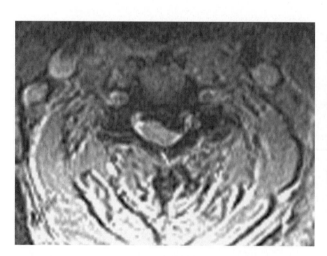

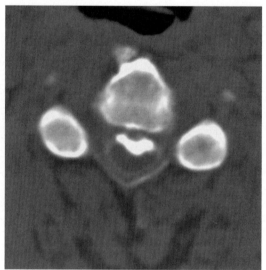

FIGURE 21.3

FIGURE 21.4

HISTORY

A 70-year-old with myelopathy.

FINDINGS

Sagittal T1-weighted (Fig. 21.1) and sagittal fast spin echo T2-weighted (Fig. 21.2) images show severe narrowing of the thecal sac spanning the C3–4, C4–5, and C5–6 levels. The linear area of abnormal low signal intensity is seen posterior to the vertebral bodies from C3 through C5–6 (*arrows*). This low signal is also present on the axial 3D-gradient echo sequence (Fig. 21.3), deforming the thecal sac and cord.

Axial CT following intrathecal contrast administration (Fig. 20.4) shows dense calcification posterior to the vertebral body, which is extradural in location, compressing the thecal sac and cord.

DIAGNOSIS

Ossification of the posterior longitudinal ligament (OPLL).

DISCUSSION

OPLL begins with calcification, followed by frank ossification of the posterior longitudinal ligament in the upper cervical spine (C3–4 or C4–5); it then progresses inferiorly to the upper thoracic spine. OPLL is shown on plain films of the cervical spine in 0.8% of asymptomatic non-Japanese Asians, 0.12% of asymptomatic North Americans, and 2.2% of the Japanese population. With clinical myelopathy, the frequency increases to 20% to 23% in the United States, and 27% in Japan. Patients tend to present in the sixth decade, generally older than the usual disk disease patient and younger than patients with cervical spondylosis. Presenting complaints include neck pain, dysesthesias, and upper- and lower-extremity weakness. Hirabayashi divided OPLL into four types based on CT: Continuous OPLL extends between vertebral bodies and crosses multiple disk spaces (27% of cases); segmental OPLL is limited to the posterior vertebral body margins (39% of cases); mixed OPLL is both continuous and segmental (29% of cases). The remaining 5% is restricted to the disk space level (21). Circumferential compression of the cord may result from combined OPLL and ossification of the ligamentum flavum. Surgical approaches include both anterior and posterior, with no clear-cut evidence to support one over the other in providing improved outcome.

In continuous OPLL, MR shows a thick band of decreased signal on T1- and T2-weighted images. Areas of increased signal may be seen within the band, which is thought to be related to marrow signal. The segmental type is more difficult to discern on MR and shows a thin area of decreased signal intensity, without signal from within the ossification region. Mass effect upon the dural sac and cord is most easily appreciated on the T2-weighted sequences.

BIBLIOGRAPHY

Baba H, Imura S, Kawahara N, et al. Diagnosis and treatment of cervical myeloradiculopathy. I. Anterior decompression and fusion for ossification of the posterior longitudinal ligament. *J Neurol Orthop Med Surg* 1993;14:79–86.

Dietemann JL, Dirheimer Y, Babin E, et al. Ossification of the posterior longitudinal ligament (Japanese disease): a radiological study in 12 cases. *J Neuroradiol* 1985;12:212–222.

Epstein NE. Ossification of the posterior longitudinal ligament: diagnosis and surgical management. *Neurosurg Q* 1992;2:223–241.

Epstein NE. The surgical management of ossification of the posterior longitudinal ligament in 51 patients. *J Spinal Disord* 1993;6:432–455.

Hirabayashi K, Watanabe K, Wakano K, et al. Expansive open door laminoplasty for cervical spinal stenotic myelopathy. *Spine* 1983;8:693–699.

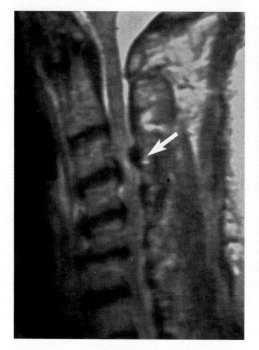

FIGURE 22.1

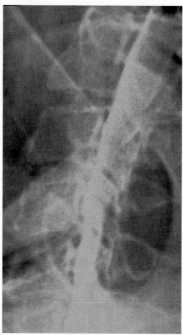

FIGURE 22.2

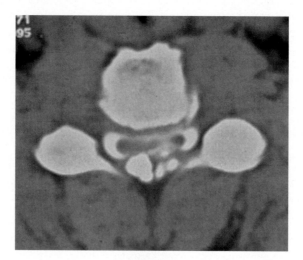

FIGURE 22.3

HISTORY

A 60-year-old with myelopathy and paresthesia.

FINDINGS

Sagittal T2-weighted fast spin echo image (Fig. 22.1) shows a rounded area of markedly diminished signal intensity, which appears extradural in location along the posterior aspect of the thecal sac at the C3–4 level (*arrow*). There is moderate bulge at the annulus fibrosis at the C3–4 as well, contributing to the severe central stenosis. Abnormal high signal intensity is present within the cervical cord at this level. A lateral view of a myelogram following intrathecal installation of contrast (Fig. 22.2) shows a long-segment extradural defect dorsal to the thecal sac at the C4 level. Axial CT image through the C4 level following intrathecal contrast administration (Fig. 22.3) shows the large globular calcifications within the ligament and flavum, which compresses the dorsal thecal sac and cord. There is marked thinning and compression of the cord by the combination of ventral and dorsal extradural disease.

DIAGNOSIS

Ossification of the ligamentum flavum with cord compression and focal myelomalacia.

DISCUSSION

Ossification of the ligamentum flavum involves formation of mature lamellar bone and is usually associated with ossification of the posterior longitudinal ligaments. Dorsal spinal cord compression secondary to ossification or calcification of the ligamentum flavum is unusual and was first described by Yamaguchi et al. It has been reported as a cause of thoracic and cervical myelopathy. Typical CT features show bilateral symmetric calcific masses centered on the ligamentum flavum, although a single central area of calcification has been reported. Magnetic resonance imaging may provide clues concerning the presence of large calcifications of the ligamentum flavum when, on T1- and T2-weighted images, a large signal void is noticed narrowing the spinal cord, compressing the sac and cord posteriorly. The lack of signal coming from the ligamentum flavum in this entity is explained by the lack of mobile protons in this calcified structure. Treatment is by excision via laminectomy. Calcium pyrophosphate deposition disease (CPPD) may show similar findings but will show positive birefringent crystals at polarized light microscopy. CPPD crystal deposition may also be seen in the ligamentum flavum associated with hyperparathyroidism, and hemochromatosis.

BIBLIOGRAPHY

Brown TR, Quinn SF, D'Agostino AN. Deposition of calcium pyrophosphate dihydrate crystals in the ligamentum flavum: evaluation with MR imaging and CT. *Radiology* 1991;178:871–873.

Hanakita J, Suwa H, Ohta F, et al. Neuroradiological examination of thoracic radiculo-myelopathy due to ossification of the ligamentum flavum. *Neuroradiology* 1990;32:38–42.

Sato R, Takahashi M, Yamashita Y, et al. Calcium crystal deposition in cervical ligamentum flavum: CT and MR findings. *J Comput Assist Tomogr* 1992;16:352–355.

Sugimura H, Kakitsubata Y, Suzuki Y, et al. MRI of ossification of ligamentum flavum. *J Comput Assist Tomogr* 1992;16:73–76.

Yamaguchi M, Tamagake S, Fujita S. A case of ossification of ligamentum flavum causing thoracic myelopathy. *J Orthop Surg* (Tokyo) 1960;11:951–956.

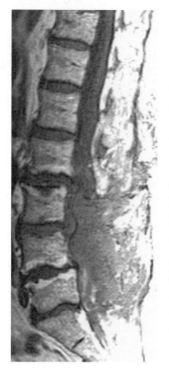 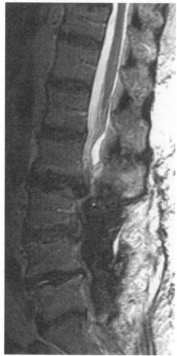 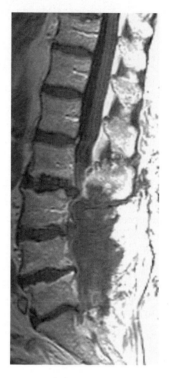

| FIGURE 23.1 | FIGURE 23.2 | FIGURE 23.3 |

HISTORY

A 49-year-old with back pain and inability to void following lumbar surgery.

FINDINGS

Sagittal T1-weighted image prior to contrast administration (Fig. 23.1) shows a wide laminectomy defect spanning L3 through L5–S1 levels. There is loss of the usual low signal intensity of the thecal sac also at this level, which merges into the posterior operative defect. Several large herniations are seen of the intervertebral disk at the L2–3 and L3–4 levels. Sagittal fast spin echo T2-weighted sequence (Fig. 23.2) demonstrates abnormal low signal intensity from the region of the thecal sac and the operative site from L3 through L5. Following contrast administration, the sagittal T1-weighted image (Fig. 23.3) shows no abnormal enhancement within this region.

DIAGNOSIS

Postoperative lumbar hematoma.

DISCUSSION

Because of the tremendous changes in the epidural soft tissues and intervertebral disk following surgery, caution must be used in MR interpretation during the first 6 weeks following surgery. There may be a large amount of tissue disruption and edema, producing mass effect on the anterior thecal sac. MR may be used in the immediate postoperative period for a more gross view of the thecal sac and epidural space, to exclude significant postoperative hemorrhage at the laminectomy site, pseudomeningocele, or disk space infection. Fat may be placed in the epidural space in an attempt to stop epidural scar formation and should not be mistaken for postoperative high signal intensity hemorrhage on T1-weighted images. A simple fat saturation technique will allow the difference to be made. Small fluid collections are not uncommonly seen in the posterior tissues following laminectomy. The signal intensities can vary somewhat, depending upon whether the collections are serous (follow CSF signal intensity) or serosanguinous (increased signal on T1-weighted images due to hemoglobin breakdown products). The distinction between small postoperative fluid collections and infected collections cannot be made by MR morphology or signal intensity. Hemorrhage typically shows iso- to increased signal in the epidural space on T1-weighted images and shows diminished signal on gradient echo or T2-weighted images. The loss of signal on T2-weighted images may be slightly minimized by the use of fast spin echo sequences, making hematoma more difficult to recognize.

BIBLIOGRAPHY

Ross JS, Masaryk TJ, Schrader M, et al. MR imaging of the postoperative lumbar spine: assessment with gadopentetate dimeglumine. *Am J Roentgenol* 1990;155:867–872.

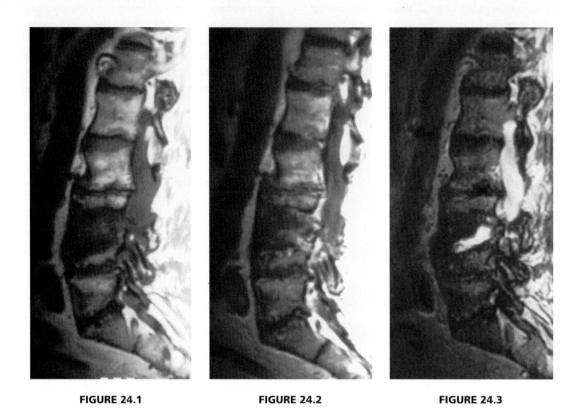

FIGURE 24.1   FIGURE 24.2   FIGURE 24.3

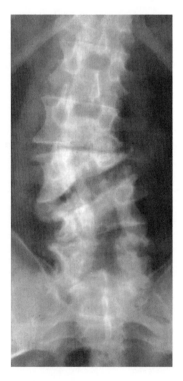

FIGURE 24.4

HISTORY

A 76-year-old with severe back pain and prior multiple surgeries.

FINDINGS

Sagittal T1-weighted image prior to contrast administration (Fig. 24.1) shows confluent low signal intensity involving the inferior aspect of L3 body and the superior aspect of L4 body and at L3–4 disk space. There is also degenerative disk disease at the levels above and below, with marked loss of disk space height. Sagittal T1 image following contrast administration (Fig. 24.2) shows a small amount of patchy enhancement within the posterior margins of these vertebral bodies and the intervertebral disk.

The bulk of the abnormal low signal seen on the unenhanced study does not show significant enhancement. Sagittal T2-weighted image (Fig. 24.3) shows an oblique area of high signal intensity involving the intervertebral disk. AP lumbar plain film (Fig. 24.4) shows an oblique lucency spanning the intervertebral disk space at L3–4 with well-defined margins and little new bony hypotrophic change. A scoliosis is associated with the deformity at the disk space level.

DIAGNOSIS

Lumbar pseudoarthrosis.

DISCUSSION

Prior surgery can produce an unstable motion segment. Biomechanical analysis has shown that the sacrifice of more than 50% of both facets or the sacrifice of one entire facet will produce significant loss of mechanical integrity. The clinical studies of this are murkier, showing acceptable clinical results even in the face of postoperative instability, as well as only a small percentage of progressive instability occurring even after extensive posterior decompressions. Many other factors undoubtedly complicate the matter of pseudoarthrosis following prior surgeries, such as age, intrinsic degenerative disease, associated osteophytes, and the particular operation involved. The association of disk excision coupled with posterior decompression may further increase the instability of the motion segment. Although fusion failure and pseudoarthrosis is a multifactorial event, in general the incidence of pseudoarthrosis is 5% following posterior surgery at one level and may be as high as 30% or greater for three or more levels of surgery. Clinical presentation of pseudoarthrosis is variable, ranging all the way from no symptomatology to disabling back pain. Pseudoarthrosis can occur along different planes. The typical pseudoarthrosis is transverse and may not only involve the posterior elements but, if there has been prior failure of anterior fusion, extend through the intervertebral disk space itself. A plate-like pseudoarthrosis occurs when the dorsal grafting material has united in a solid fashion, but it is separate from the underlying laminae and transverse processes.

In this instance, the pseudoarthrosis must be distinguished from disk space infection or severe degenerative disease. Although there is loss of end plate and disk definition (which can be seen with disk space infection), there is no exuberant or abundant enhancement to suggest a more aggressive process such as disk space infection. Additional entities to include in a differential are neurotrophic or Charcot joint, or a more indolent infection such as tuberculosis or fungi.

BIBLIOGRAPHY

Eschelman DJ, Beers GJ, Naimark A, et al. Pseudoarthrosis in ankylosing spondylitis mimicking infectious diskitis: MR appearance. *Am J Neuroradiol* 1991;12:1113.

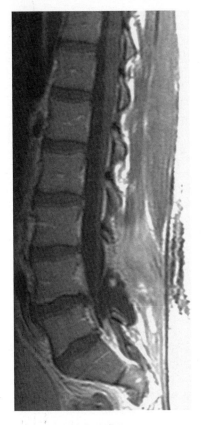

FIGURE 25.1

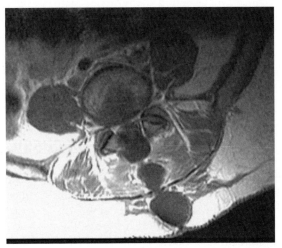

FIGURE 25.2

HISTORY

A 46-year-old with low back discomfort following surgery.

FINDINGS

Sagittal (Fig. 25.1) and axial (Fig. 25.2) T1-weighted images following contrast administration show a laminectomy defect at the L4 and L5 levels. A well-defined lobulated collection mimicking CSF signal intensity extends along the dorsal operative tract into the subcutaneous tissues. No intrinsic enhancement is seen. There is a small disk protrusion at L4–5 with no evidence of thecal sac compromise.

DIAGNOSIS

Pseudomeningocele.

DISCUSSION

A pseudomeningocele results from a dural tear at the time of surgery. MR imaging in these cases will show a rounded area of CSF signal intensity posterior to the thecal sac at the site of previous laminectomy, and CT will show CSF attenuation. An intermediate-signal-intensity fibrous capsule may be present. Fluid-fluid levels may be seen in these collections due to layering of debris or blood products. Although the fluid collection itself is readily identified, the precise location of the tear cannot be defined. The differential would include postoperative serous fluid collections, which are not uncommonly present after surgery, and infected collections. There are no signal-intensity differences between the fluid collections. Similar findings can be identified with CT myelography, with contrast filling the fluid collection.

BIBLIOGRAPHY

Ross JS, Masaryk TJ, Schrader M, et al. MR imaging of the postoperative lumbar spine: assessment with gadopentetate dimeglumine. *Am J Roentgenol* 1990;155:867–872.

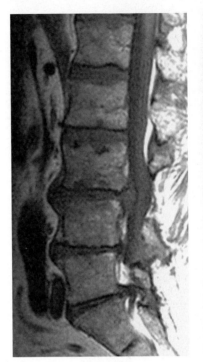

FIGURE 26.1

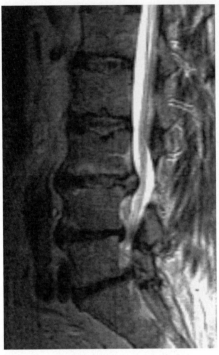

FIGURE 26.2

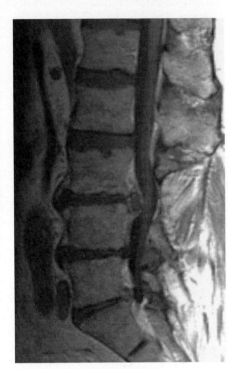

FIGURE 26.3

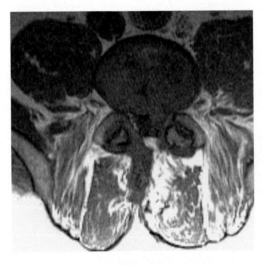

FIGURE 26.4

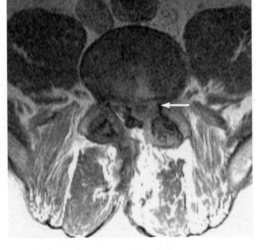

FIGURE 26.5

HISTORY

A 52-year-old with left lower-extremity pain extending below the knee. The patient had L3–4 laminectomy and diskectomy 3 years ago.

FINDINGS

Sagittal T1 (Fig. 26.1) and sagittal fast spin echo T2 (Fig. 26.2) images show a soft-tissue lesion at the L3–4 level within the anterior epidural space and contiguous with the L3–4 disk space. This shows a well-defined posterior margin. Following contrast administration (Fig. 26.3) the sagittal T1-weighted image shows central area that does not enhance with peripheral enhancement. The peripheral enhancement is confirmed when viewed by the axial T1-weighted image without contrast (Fig. 26.4) and with contrast (Fig. 26.5) (*arrow*).

DIAGNOSIS

Disk herniation and epidural fibrosis.

DISCUSSION

The use of Gd-DTPA-enhanced MR in the evaluation of scar versus disk has been examined by Hueftle et al. Thirty patients were evaluated with MR before and after administration of Gd-DTPA (0.1 mmol/kg body weight), with repeat surgery in 17 patients. Enhanced MR correctly predicted the surgical findings in all 17 patients. The findings may be divided into three categories: scar only, disk only, and scar plus disk. Scar tissue consistently was seen to enhance immediately following injection, regardless of the time since surgery. Epidural scar has been seen to enhance in patients who had surgery more than 20 years earlier. Scar tissue occasionally shows mass effect. Therefore this finding should not be used as a major discriminator of disk versus scar. Disk material does not enhance on the early postinjection images because of its avascular nature. If images are obtained longer than 30 minutes after injection, however, disk material may enhance because of diffusion of contrast into the disk from adjacent vascularized tissue. In patients with a mixture of scar and disk material, scar enhances and the disk material does not enhance on early postinjection images. However, the disk material consistently enhances if enough time is allowed for diffusion of contrast into the disk material from the surrounding vascular scar. Similar findings have been noted using iodinated contrast material with CT. Two points must be mentioned about this technique. First, one must obtain both sagittal and T1-weighted images before and after administration of contrast. Ideally, the patient should not be moved between the scans taken before and after contrast administration to ensure precise comparison between the same regions of interest. Second, one must complete the postinjection images within the first 20 minutes following contrast administration. Ross et al. updated the numbers in this series, with an additional 27 patients undergoing repeat surgery following contrast-enhanced MR, with a 96% accuracy in differentiating scar from disk in 44 patients and 50 levels.

Problems might occur when the volume of nonenhancing herniated disk is small relative to the volume of enhancing scar tissue, in which case partial volume averaging might obscure the disk. Additionally, when scar tissue invades the disk material as part of the body's reparative process, the disk material might show enhancement. Overall, 6 weeks or more after surgery, sagittal and axial T1-weighted pre- and post-Gd-DTPA MR remains the most effective method of evaluating the postoperative patient with lumbar spine disease. Selective fat suppression has been used in the evaluation of the postoperative patients. Georgy examined 25 patients with recurrent pain after lumbar disk surgery with MR to evaluate the usefulness of contrast-enhanced fat-suppression imaging in patients with failed back surgery. The addition of fat suppression to Gd-enhanced T1-weighted images improved the visualization of enhancing scar in all of their cases, helped distinguish scar from recurrent herniated disk, and showed more clearly the relationship of scar to the nerve roots and thecal sac. They recommend the combination of unenhanced and Gd-enhanced T1-weighted images with fat suppression for routine examination of the postoperative back.

BIBLIOGRAPHY

Georgy BA, Hesselink JR, Middleton MS. Fat suppression contrast-enhanced MRI in the failed back surgery syndrome: a prospective study. *Neuroradiology* 1995;37:51–57.

Hochhauser L, Kieffer SA, Cacayorin ED, et al. Recurrent postdiskectomy low back pain: MR-surgical correlation. *Am J Roentgenol* 1988;151:755–760.

Hueftle MG, Modic MT, Ross JS, et al. Lumbar spine: postoperative MR imaging with Gd-DTPA. *Radiology* 1988;167:817.

Ross JS. Magnetic resonance imaging of the postoperative spine. *Top Magn Reson Imaging* 1988;1:39–52.

Ross JS. The postoperative lumbar spine. *Semin Spine Surg* 1997;9:28–37.

Ross JS, Delamarter R, Hueftle MG, et al. Gadolinium-DTPA-enhanced MR imaging of the postoperative lumbar spine: time course and mechanism of enhancement. *Am J Roentgenol* 1989;152:825–834.

Sotiropoulos S, Chafetz NI, Lang P, et al. Differentiation between postoperative scar and recurrent disk herniation: prospective comparison of MR, CT, and contrast-enhanced CT. *Am J Neuroradiol* 1989;10:639–643.

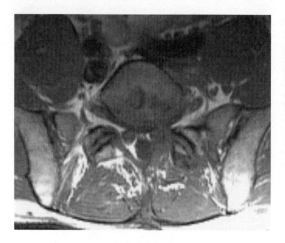

FIGURE 27.1

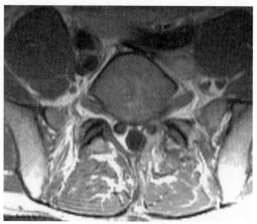

FIGURE 27.2

HISTORY

A 36-year-old with left leg pain and a history of prior L5–S1 laminectomy and diskectomy.

FINDINGS

Axial T1-weighted image at the L5–S1 level without contrast (Fig. 27.1) and with contrast (Fig. 27.2) show homogeneous soft tissue along the left lateral aspect of the thecal sac and surrounding and exiting the S1 root. This demonstrates homogeneous enhancement following contrast administration.

DIAGNOSIS

Epidural fibrosis.

DISCUSSION

Lumbar peridural fibrosis (scar) is a replacement of the normal epidural fat with postoperative fibrotic tissue, which is capable of binding the dura and nerve roots to the surrounding structures anteriorly and posteriorly. Peridural scar formation has never been directly proven to cause postoperative radicular and/or low back pain. Nevertheless, postoperative peridural fibrosis has been attributed by a number of clinical investigators as one of the major causes of recurrent radicular and/or low back pain after lumbar laminectomy and diskectomy. These reports do not directly link peridural fibrosis with recurrent pain and tend to be retrospective, with small patient numbers and without modern imaging correlation of the presence of epidural fibrosis such as MR. Despite the lack of direct proof of the symptom-producing nature of peridural fibrosis, a large amount of literature has been devoted to experimental studies designed to decrease

the amount of scar or to keep scar from forming dense adhesions to the dura. A variety of materials, including silastic Dacron, methacrylate, bone graft, synthetic membranes and foams, free and pedicle fat grafts, carboxymethylcellulose, elastase, and sodium hyaluronate have been evaluated in an effort to stop or limit peridural fibrosis. A recent report describes 197 patients who underwent first-time single-level unilateral diskectomy for lumbar disk herniation and were evaluated in a randomized, double-blind, controlled, multicenter clinical trial that demonstrated that there is a significant association between the presence of extensive peridural scar and the occurrence of recurrent radicular pain. Clinical assessments were conducted preoperatively and at 1 and 6 months postoperatively, and enhanced MR images were obtained at 6 months postoperatively. Radicular pain was recorded by the patient using a validated visual analog pain scale in which 0 equals no pain and 10 equals excruciating pain. The data obtained at the 6-month time point were analyzed for an association between amount of peridural scar as measured by MR imaging and clinical failure as defined by the recurrence of radicular pain. The results showed that probability of recurrent pain increases when scar score increases. Patients having extensive peridural scar were 3.2 times more likely to experience recurrent radicular pain than those with less extensive peridural scarring.

Epidural fibrosis is seen to consistently enhance immediately following injection of contrast material. This enhancement occurs regardless of the time since surgery. Epidural scar has been seen to enhance in patients whose surgery was more than 20 years ago, so time since surgery should not dissuade one from using contrast material in the postoperative state. Scar tissue did occasionally show mass effect and should not be used as the major discriminator of disk versus scar. Disk material does not enhance on the early postinjection images because it is avascular. However, if delayed images are obtained (greater than 20 to 30 minutes following injection), then disk material may enhance due to diffusion of contrast into the disk from adjacent vascularized scar tissue. In those cases with a mixture of scar and disk material, scar will enhance and the disk material will not enhance on early postinjection images. However, the disk material will consistently enhance if enough time is given for diffusion of contrast into the disk material from the surrounding vascular scar.

BIBLIOGRAPHY

Bundschuh CV, Modic MT, Ross JS, et al. Epidural fibrosis and recurrent disk herniation in the lumbar spine: MR imaging assessment. *Am J Neuroradiol* 1988;9:169–178.

Bundschuh CV, Stein L, Slusser JH, et al. Distinguishing between scar and recurrent herniated disk in postoperative patients: value of contrast-enhanced CT and MR imaging. *Am J Neuroradiol* 1990;11:949–958.

Ross JS, Delamarter R, Hueftle MG, et al. Gadolinium-DTPA-enhanced MR imaging of the postoperative lumbar spine: time course and mechanism of enhancement. *Am J Roentgenol* 1989;152:825–834.

Ross JS, Frederickson RCA, Petrie JL, et al. Association between peridural scar and recurrent radicular pain after lumbar discectomy: MR evaluation. *Neurosurgery* 1996;38:855–863.

Ross JS. Magnetic resonance imaging of the postoperative spine. *Top Magn Reson Imaging* 1988;1:39–52.

Ross JS. The postoperative lumbar spine. *Semin Spine Surg* 1997;9:28–37.

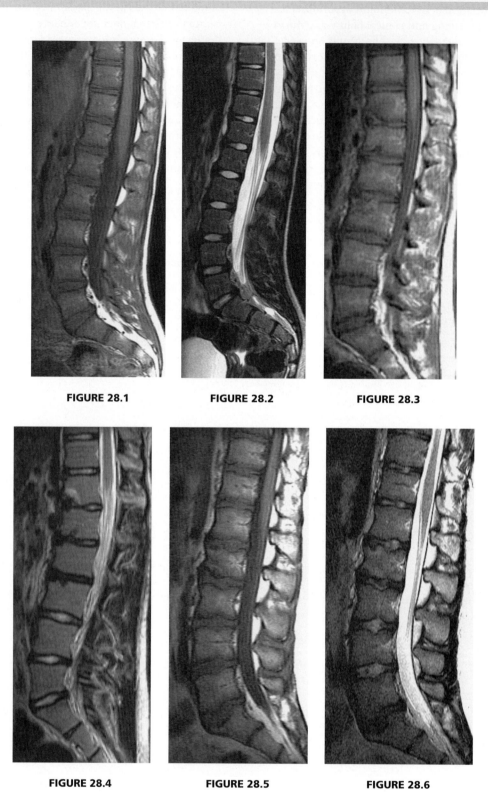

FIGURE 28.1　　**FIGURE 28.2**　　**FIGURE 28.3**

FIGURE 28.4　　**FIGURE 28.5**　　**FIGURE 28.6**

HISTORY

Two teenagers with back pain. A normal is shown for comparison purposes.

FINDINGS

Two abnormal cases are presented, with a normal adolescent spine on T1-weighted sagittal (Fig. 28.1) and fast spin echo T2-weighted (Fig. 28.2) shown for comparison purposes. In the first abnormal case, the sagittal T1 (Fig. 28.3) and sagittal T2 fast spin echo (Fig. 28.4) show loss of the usual lumbar lordosis. There is loss of disk space height and signal intensity on T2-weighted images at the T12–L1 through L2–3 levels. End-plate irregularities are noted at multiple levels as well. No definite disk protrusion is seen. In the second patient, the sagittal T1-weighted image (Fig. 28.5) and the sagittal T2-weighted image (Fig. 28.6) show degeneration, with loss of disk space height at several levels as well as multiple end-plate irregularities extending from L1 through L5–S1 levels.

DIAGNOSIS

Scheuermann's disease.

DISCUSSION

The most common causes of serious low-back pain in children are spondylolysis, Scheuermann's disease, and muscular ligamentous injury. Scheuermann's disease has been known by a variety of terms, including *spinal osteochondrosis, kyphosis dorsalis juvenilis, Scheuermann's juvenile kyphosis,* and *vertebral epiphysitis.* The classic description for Scheuermann's disease involves a progressive thoracic kyphosis in an adolescent or young adult, associated with at least three abnormal-appearing and wedge-shaped vertebral bodies and/or three levels of end-plate irregularity (Schmorl's nodes). This was initially thought to represent a vertebral inflammatory epiphysitis but is now considered a manifestation of degenerative disk disease. Various radiographic features have been described, including an increased AP diameter to the vertebral body, wedge-shaped vertebral body, narrow disk spaces, kyphosis or loss of lordosis, Schmorl's nodes, and detached epiphyseal rings. Changes usually affect the lower thoracic or upper lumbar vertebral bodies; however, multiple bodies can be involved. No precise pathologic mechanism is known, although the current concept involves collagen weakness in the vertebral end plates, leading to abnormally soft bodies that become wedged and susceptible to end-plate herniations (Schmorl's nodes). Wedging of the anterior portions of the vertebral bodies with marked kyphotic deformity allows the diagnosis of classic Scheuermann's disease. However, this can also occur in the lumbar spine and must be considered in a young patient with evidence of irregularity of the end plate, Schmorl's nodes, and diminished disk space without wedging. In general, the prognosis is good, with progression of curved abnormalities in both the typical and atypical types being uncommon. Progression can occur and follow-up may be necessary. In general, the prognosis for those exhibiting Scheuermann's disease in the thoracic area is good, moderately good for those of the thoracolumbar area, and worst for the lumbar spine with regard to work capacity. The appearance of end-plate irregularity in Schmorl's nodes is common within the population, and some have estimated that Scheuermann's disease affects nearly 10% of the population. Only 1%, however, ever seek medical attention during their youth.

For comparison in this case we provide T1- and T2-weighted images of a normal adolescent spine. In each of the two cases, the Scheuermann's disease is manifest by evidence of degeneration, loss of disk space height, loss of signal intensity on T2-weighted images, and multiple end-plate irregularities.

BIBLIOGRAPHY

Paajanen H, Erkintalo M, Kuusela T, et al. Magnetic resonance study of disc degeneration in young low-back pain patients. *Spine* 1989;14:982–985.

Salminen JJ, Erkintalo TM, Paajanen HK. Magnetic resonance imaging findings of lumbar spine in the young: correlation with leisure time physical activity, spinal mobility, and trunk muscle strength in 15-year-old pupils with or without low-back pain. *J Spinal Disord* 1993;6:386–391.

Tertti MO, Salminen JJ, Paajanen HK, et al. Low-back pain and disk degeneration in children: a case-control MR imaging study. *Radiology* 1991;180:503–507.

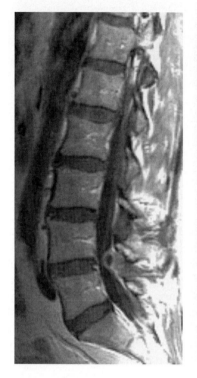

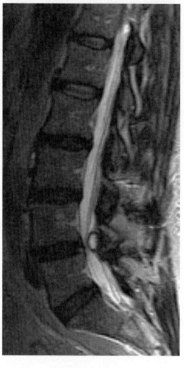

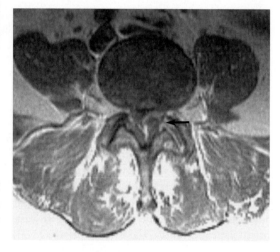

| **FIGURE 29.1** | **FIGURE 29.2** | **FIGURE 29.3** |

HISTORY

A 48-year-old with left leg radiculopathy.

FINDINGS

Sagittal T1-weighted image following contrast (Fig. 29.1) and sagittal fast spin echo T2-weighted image (Fig. 29.2) show a well-defined rounded lesion involving the dorsal epidural space at the L4–5 level. This shows peripheral enhancement and is strikingly low in signal intensity on the T2-weighted sequence. Axial image following contrast administration (Fig. 29.3) confirms the dorsal lateral epidural location and adjacent to the facet joint (*arrow*).

DIAGNOSIS

Synovial cyst.

DISCUSSION

Synovial cysts are associated with degenerative changes of the facet joints and may cause mass effect on the thecal sac and radiculopathy. The imaging features include a relatively low-signal lesion centered just anterior and medial to the anterior facet margin, with posterolateral mass effect on the thecal sac. With larger lesions the direction of mass effect may not be apparent. T2-weighted images are helpful because they show increased signal, similar to CSF from the central portion of the lesion. Contrast administration can turn a difficult diagnosis into an easy one. With contrast, the synovial cyst shows well-defined peripheral enhancement, with the posterior margin abutting against the degenerated facet joint. The lesions tend to be very difficult to define on T1-weighted images, making fast spin echo T2- or contrast-enhanced T1 images necessary. The differential is limited, and with larger lesions a cystic Schwannoma is a possibility. These lesions usually have more irregular enhancement, however. (See Case 70.)

BIBLIOGRAPHY

Caputo N, Lucciolo R, Castrioto C, et al. Synovial cyst of the ligamentum flavum of the lumbar canal: description of a case. *Riv Neurobiol* 1989;18:71–73.

Davis R, Iliya A, Roque C, et al. The advantage of magnetic resonance imaging in diagnosis of a lumbar synovial cyst. *Spine* 1990;15:244–246.

Fletcher EE, Scott WR. Lumbar synovial cysts: report of eleven cases. *Neurosurgery* 1989;24:112–115.

Jackson-DE J, Atlas SW, Mani JR, et al. Intraspinal synovial cysts: MR imaging. *Radiology* 1989;170:527–530.

Liu SS, Williams KD, Drayer BP, et al. Synovial cysts of the lumbosacral spine: diagnosis by MR imaging. *Am J Neuroradiol* 1989;10:1239–1242.

Rosenblum J, Mojtahedi S, Fopust RJ. Synovial cysts in the lumbar spine: MR characteristics. *Am J Neuroradiol* 1989;10:S94.

Silbergleit R, Gebarski SS, Brunberg JA, et al. Lumbar synovial cysts: correlation of myelographic, CT, MR, and pathologic findings. *Am J Neuroradiol* 1990;11:777–779.

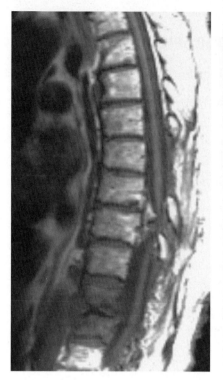

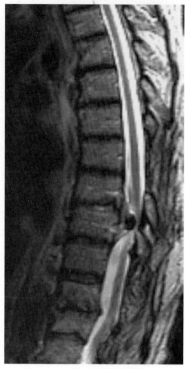

FIGURE 30.1   FIGURE 30.2

HISTORY

A 72-year-old with spastic leg weakness progressing over the last 10 months.

FINDINGS

Sagittal T1-weighted (Fig. 30.1) and sagittal fast spin echo T2-weighted (Fig. 30.2) images of the thoracic spine demonstrate a large extradural lesion anteriorly that shows predominantly low signal on the T2 image and areas of high signal on the T1-weighted images. This is a broad-based margin. It is centered about an intervertebral disk level. There is compression of the thecal sac and cord due to the anterior extradural mass. There is incidental marked degenerative change at the thoracolumbar junction with low signal on the T1-weighted images within the two adjacent vertebral bodies, showing high signal on T2 due to type I degenerative end-plate change. Vacuum phenomena are also present at that lower thoracolumbar level.

DIAGNOSIS

Ossified thoracic disk herniation.

DISCUSSION

Thoracic disk herniations have been difficult to diagnosis and to treat, with a myriad of potential surgical approaches and clinical presentations. MR has made the diagnosis much easier, with its increased sensitivity to thoracic herniations and ability to diagnose minimal or asymptomatic disk herniations. Surgical treatment for herniated thoracic disks is uncommon and reflects approximately 4% of all disk operations. Treatment has been difficult, which has been related to diagnostic delays, and indications for surgery have been poor. Presence of severe or progressive myelopathy is generally regarded as an absolute indication for surgery. The annual incidence of thoracic herniations causing neurologic deficits is one per 1 million population. However, 15% to 20% of the population may have incidental thoracic disk herniations visible on MR images.

MR is not without its problems, which includes the inability to distinguish areas of calcification, which may change surgical approach; potential overestimation of degree of mass effect on the cord; and possibility of imprecisely localizing the level of abnormality, if definitive scout views are not performed. There is also little consensus on indications for disk removal and considerable variability in the surgical approaches. Historically, laminectomy has given disappointing results. Posterolateral surgeries such as transpedicular and transfacet pedicle-sparing approaches are considered by many as simpler operations than their anterolateral and lateral counterparts. The anterolateral approaches include transthoracic, thoracoscopic, and retropleural thoracotomy; lateral approaches include costotransversectomy and parascapular. Stillerman proposed the following management scheme:

1. Patients with localized or axial pain without myelopathy are not surgically treated. They are treated conservatively with steroids or nonsteroidal antiinflammatories and physical therapy.
2. Patients with radiculopathy alone have medical treatment, with occasional steroid injections into the intercostal nerve. Patients with persistent radicular complaints who do not improve are evaluated for surgery, which may consist of the posterolateral approach.
3. If imaging reveals large herniation with myelopathy, then treatment is based on the status of the neurologic deficit. When myelopathy is progressive or severe, patients are put into a high- or low-risk category. If in a low-risk category, patients with lateral herniations have posterolateral surgery. Calcification also may modify this approach. High-risk medical patients with densely calcified central herniations are treated conservatively.

BIBLIOGRAPHY

Brown CW, Deffer-PA J, Akmakjian J, et al. The natural history of thoracic disc herniation. *Spine* 1992;17:S97–S102.
Chin LS, Black KL, Hoff JT. Multiple thoracic disc herniations: case report. *J Neurosurg* 1987;66:290–292.
Ross JS, Perez RN, Masaryk TJ, et al. Thoracic disk herniation: MR imaging. *Radiology* 1987;165:511–515.
Stillerman CB, Chen TC, Couldwell WT, et al. Experience in the surgical management of 82 symptomatic herniated thoracic discs and review of the literature. *J Neurosurg* 1998;88:623–633.

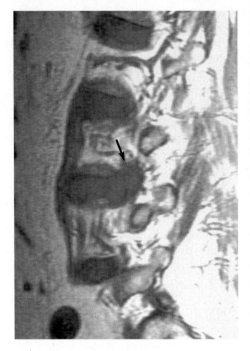

FIGURE 31.1

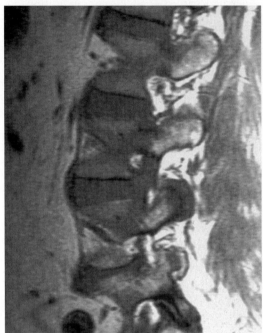

FIGURE 31.2

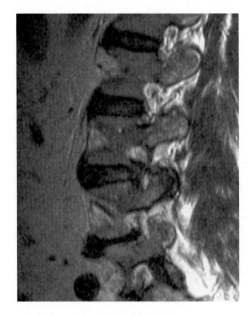

FIGURE 31.3

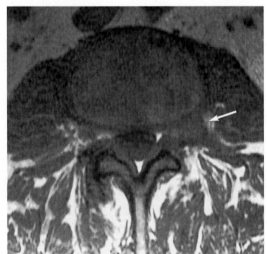

FIGURE 31.4

HISTORY

A 39-year-old with right leg pain.

FINDINGS

Left parasagittal T1-weighted images (Figs. 31.1 and 31.2) show a well-defined mass arising from the level of the disk at the L4–5 level and extending into the inferior portion of the neural foramen (*arrow*). The sagittal T2-weighted image (Fig. 31.3) shows the mass tracking the signal intensity of the intervertebral disk. The axial T1-weighted image (Fig. 31.4) demonstrates the contiguity of the left lateral and intraforaminal mass with the disk margin and the extension into the region of the left L4 ganglion.

DIAGNOSIS

Lateral lumbar disk herniation.

DISCUSSION

Foraminal disk herniations occur in 3% to 10% of all disk herniations. They may reside within the foramen or laterally and be extraforaminal. They compress the exiting root at that level (i.e., an L4–5 herniation will compress the L4 root). This is in contrast to the classic pattern of a more central or lateral herniation that occurs inferior to the root at that level and compresses the level below (i.e., an L4–5 central herniation compressing the L5 root). Most of these herniations occur at L3–4 and L4–5 levels and are found in older patients. Pain onset may be sudden and the patient may present with severe anterior thigh pain. Surgical approach is varied but may involve an interlaminar window (with loss of facet), or more likely, an extraforaminal posterolateral approach.

On MR, the findings are a soft-tissue mass tracking the usual disk signal intensity that is contiguous with apparent disk space. Differential is primarily one of schwannoma, and in that case contrast administration will help. Schwannomas would be expected to enhance more homogeneously, whereas the disk herniation will show typical peripheral enhancement in the central nonenhancing area. T2 signal may also help, and if it is low in signal then it is more typical of herniation than schwannoma.

BIBLIOGRAPHY

Osborne AG, Hood RS, Sherry RG, et al. CT/MR spectrum of far lateral and anterior lumbosacral disc herniations. *Am J Neuroradiol* 1988;9:775–778.

Postacchini F, Cinotti G, Gumina S. Microsurgical excision of lateral lumbar disc herniation through an interlaminar approach. *J Bone Joint Surg Br* 1998;80:201–207.

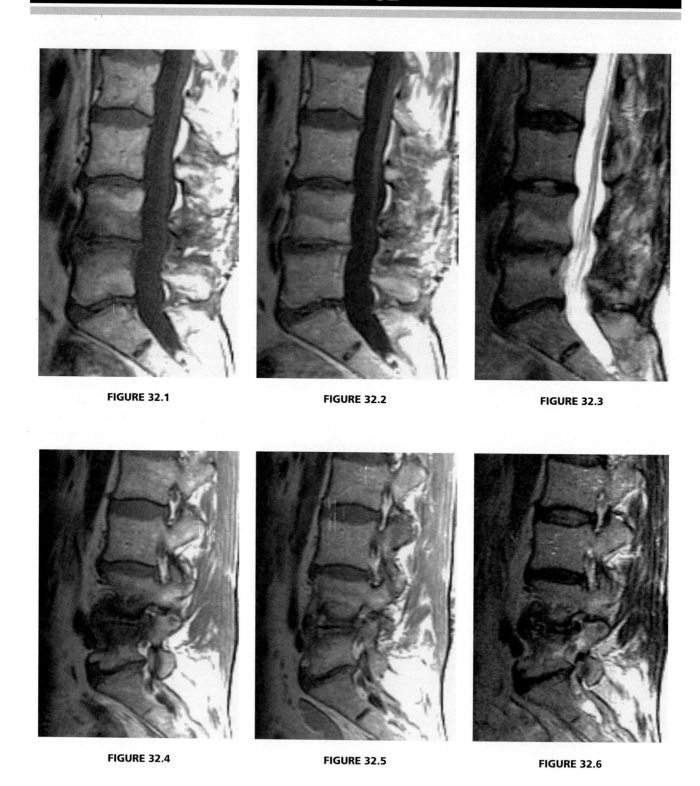

FIGURE 32.1

FIGURE 32.2

FIGURE 32.3

FIGURE 32.4

FIGURE 32.5

FIGURE 32.6

HISTORY

A 46-year-old with generalized low back pain and no other constitutional symptoms, such as fever or malaise.

FINDINGS

Sagittal T1-weighted image without contrast (Fig. 32.1), sagittal T1-weighted image following contrast (Fig. 32.2), and fast spin echo T2-weighted image (Fig. 32.3) in the midline demonstrate loss of disk space height at the L3–4, L4–5, and L5–S1 levels. There is also diminished signal intensity within these disks at L4–5 and L5–S1 on the T2-weighted sequence. Linear low signal intensity within these three disks that can reflect vacuum phenomena/calcification. Parallel bands of low signal intensity present at L4–5

bodies on the unenhanced image that show contrast enhancement and high signal on the T2-weighted image. The more paraspinal views in the same patient demonstrate on the unenhanced T1-weighted image (Fig. 32.4) low signal intensity of the adjacent L4–5 bodies. Following contrast (Fig. 32.5), there is mild and patchy enhancement but no intervertebral disk enhancement. Sagittal T2-weighted images in a parasagittal location (Fig. 32.6) showed diminished signal intensity from the adjacent vertebral body end plates.

DIAGNOSIS

Type I/III degenerative end-plate change.

DISCUSSION

MR is sensitive to marrow disease, and degenerative disk disease is no exception. Three major types of marrow in end-plate changes have been described with MR. In type I changes the vertebral bodies paralleling the end plates and degenerated disk show decreased signal intensity on T1-weighted images and increased signal intensity on T2-weighted images. These changes have been noted in approximately 4% of patients undergoing MR for lumbar disease. Type I changes have also been seen after patients have undergone chymopapain injection into disks, which can be viewed as a model of accelerated disk degeneration. At histology, type I changes show replacement of normal, fatty, cellular vertebral body marrow by fibrovascular marrow with greater water content, which prolongs both the T1 and the T2. Type I end plates also enhance following injection of Gd-DTPA, again reflecting the vascularity of the fibrous marrow changes.

Type II changes are manifested by increased signal intensity on T1-weighted images and an isointense to slightly increased signal intensity on T2-weighted images. These changes have been seen in 16% of patients undergoing MR of the lumbar spine. At histology the type II changes show

evidence of end-plate disruption, with yellow marrow replacement in the adjacent vertebral body. Types I and II changes are always seen in conjunction with evidence of disk degeneration. Type I changes have been seen to convert to type II changes with time, whereas type II changes seem to be more stable. It is currently unknown why these changes occur or if they are symptomatic.

Type III end-plate changes show decreased signal intensity on T1- and T2-weighted images and correlate with extensive bony sclerosis on plain films. Types I and II changes do not correlate with plain-film findings.

Occasionally, type I changes may be difficult to distinguish from disk space infection. In the adult population the critical factor is the appearance of the intervertebral disk. With infection the disk shows an abnormally increased signal intensity on T2-weighted images in an abnormal configuration. Usually, type I changes are associated with disks of low signal intensity because of the severe degenerative disease. However, occasionally the degenerative process forms cysts within the degenerated disk, which can be high in signal intensity on T2-weighted images and thus impossible to differentiate from infection.

BIBLIOGRAPHY

De Roos RA, Kressel H, Spritzer C, et al. MR imaging of marrow changes adjacent to end plates in degenerative lumbar disk disease. *Am J Roentgenol* 1987;149:531–534.

Modic MT, Steinberg PM, Ross JS, et al. Degenerative disk disease: assessment of changes in vertebral body marrow with MR imaging. *Radiology* 1988;166:193–199.

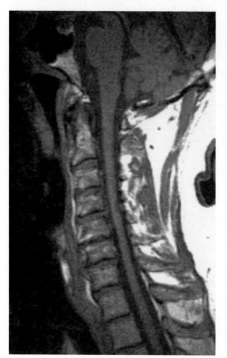

FIGURE 33.1

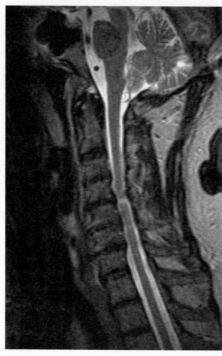

FIGURE 33.2

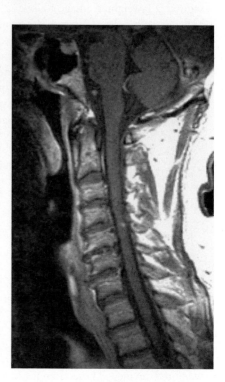

FIGURE 33.3

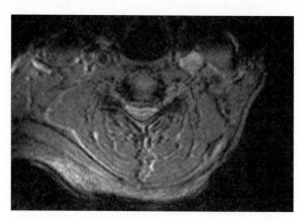

FIGURE 33.4

HISTORY

A 54-year-old with myelopathy.

FINDINGS

Sagittal T1-weighted (Fig. 33.1), sagittal fast spin echo T2-weighted (Fig. 33.2) and sagittal T1-weighted images following contrast administration (Fig. 33.3) demonstrate severe canal stenosis at the C4–5 level due to dorsal ligamentous hypertrophy as well as broad-based bulging of the annulus fibrosis anteriorly. Focal high signal is seen within the cervical cord on the T2-weighted image at the C4–5 level, which also demonstrates enhancement following contrast administration. Axial gradient echo image (Fig. 33.4) confirms the severe degree of canal stenosis and linear high signal intensity within the cord.

DIAGNOSIS

Cervical cord contusion in cervical spondylosis

DISCUSSION

The pathogenesis of cervical spondylotic myelopathy relates to cord impression from multiple ideologies relating to degenerative disease. These include the osseous and soft-tissue structure surrounding the cord, disk degeneration with bulge and/or herniation, and hyperostosis with spondylotic bars. These bars are referred to by several names, including *osteophytes* and *chondroosseous spurs*. As degenerative disk disease occurs and there is loss of disk space height there can be overriding of the uncovertebral joints. Degenerative osteoarthritis of the facet joints produces hypertrophic spurring that can contribute to canal and foraminal narrowing. Finally, the ligament flavum can hypertrophy and invaginate and contribute to canal narrowing in the cervical spine as it does in central stenosis involving the lumbar spine.

General guidelines for surgical intervention include progressive neurologic deterioration, hopefully being performed on the patient with early myelopathic findings. One difficult aspect of assessing surgical outcome is that there are no randomized studies comparing operative and nonoperative outcomes in this patient population. A study by Lesoin showed that only 10% of patients had deterioration following surgery over a 20-year period, whereas in those patients having nonoperative management, 64% had no improvement and 26% deteriorated. An additional study by Epstein et al. showed 69% of patients had improvement following surgery. Concerning specific types of surgery, no major differences between the results have been shown regarding anterior-posterior approaches for the treatment of cervical spondylotic myelopathy. Anterior approaches can be divided into anterior inner-body arthrodesis and anterior corpectomies. The anterior approach is medial to the sternocleidomastoid muscle and the carotid artery and lateral to the trachea and esophagus. The disk(s) under direct vision are removed in their entirety (in contrast to the type of removal present at lumbar laminectomy and diskectomy). The end plates are curetted and the iliac crest graft is placed with manual distraction of the disk space. The osteophytes may or may not be removed. Effectiveness of this type of surgery is limited if more than three disk levels are involved. In the anterior corpectomy, the disks are removed and a vertebrectomy or corpectomy is performed in the midline. The spinal cord is fully decompressed, but the lateral vertebral body is left, which supports the graft. The graft is placed into a trough that is produced in the end vertebral bodies. This type of surgery is performed to provide a more direct and extensive access to the spinal cord, and is generally the choice for cervical spondylotic myelopathy with deformity. The posterior approaches consist of laminectomy and open-door laminaplasties. Laminectomies are generally recommended for compression of the cord at multiple levels (three or more). These can include foraminotomies if there is also a radiculopathy component to the symptoms. Up to 50% of the facets may be removed without producing instability in the spine. Open-door laminaplasty expands the canal by lifting the lamina en bloc on one hinge. This type of surgery was initially described for treatment of cord compression due to ossification of the posterior longitudinal ligament. Rowland presents a comprehensive view of the controversies surrounding the treatment and outcome of cervical spondylotic myelopathy.

Routine MR imaging for cervical spondylosis includes sagittal T1- and T2- (or fast T2-) weighted images, and axial imaging with either two-dimensional or three-dimensional low-flip angle gradient echo images to provide high-signal-intensity CSF. Contrast administration is useful if signal or contour abnormality is detected within the cord. Takahashi et al. and others have described areas of increased signal intensity on T2-weighted images within the cervical cord due to extradural compression, which variously reflects myelomalacia, gliosis, and demyelination and edema. Patients who show areas of abnormal signal within the cord tend to have a worse clinical condition than those with normal cord signal intensity. Further, these abnormal signal changes can disappear or diminish following surgery.

BIBLIOGRAPHY

Epstein JA, Janin Y, Carras R, et al. A comparative study of the treatment of cervical spondylotic myeloradiculopathy. Experience with 50 cases treated by means of extensive laminectomy, foraminotomy, and excision of osteophytes during the past 10 years. *Acta Neurochir* 1982;61:89–104.

Haupts M, Haan J. Further aspects of MR-signal enhancements in stenosis of the cervical spinal canal: MRI investigations in correlation to clinical and CSF findings. *Neuroradiology* 1988;30:545–546.

Hirabayashi K, Miyakawa J, Satomi K, et al. Operative results and postoperative progression of ossification among patients with ossification of cervical posterior longitudinal ligament. *Spine* 1981;6:354–364.

Lesoin F, Bouasakao N, Clarisse J, et al. Results of surgical treatment of radiculomyelopathy caused by cervical arthrosis based on 1000 operations. *Surg Neurol* 1985;23:350–355.

Matsuda Y, Miyazaki K, Tada K, et al. Increased MR signal intensity due to cervical myelopathy: analysis of 29 surgical cases. *J Neurosurg* 1991;74:887–892.

Raynor RB, Pugh J, Shapiro I. Cervical facetectomy and its effects on spine strength. *J Neurosurg* 1985;63:278–282.

Rowland LP. Surgical treatment of cervical spondylotic myelopathy: time for a controlled trial. *Neurology* 1992;42:5–13.

Takahashi M, Sakamoto Y, Miyawaki M, et al. Increased MR signal intensity secondary to chronic cervical cord compression. *Neuroradiology* 1987;29:550–556.

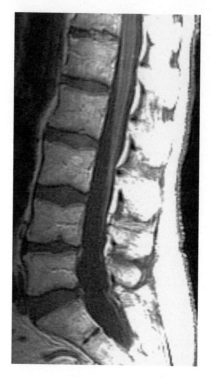

FIGURE 34.1

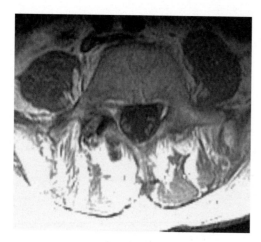

FIGURE 34.2

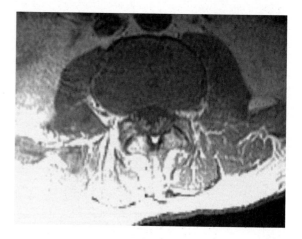

FIGURE 34.3

HISTORY

A 40-year-old following renal transplant, now with paresthesias and fever.

FINDINGS

Sagittal T1-weighted (Fig. 34.1) and two axial T1-weighted images (Figs. 34.2 and 34.3) through the lumbar spine following contrast administration show moderate leptomeningeal enhancement along the conus and the cauda equina in a diffuse fashion. No intradural masses are seen. Mild degenerative disease is noted at L4–5 and L5–S1, with no evidence of thecal sac compromise. Degenerative enhancement is also seen within the T12–L1 intervertebral disk.

DIAGNOSIS

Aspergillus meningitis.

DISCUSSION

Aspergillus species are ubiquitous, and the most common human pathogens are *Aspergillus fumigates* and *A. flavus*. Infection can occur when aspergillus is inhaled into the upper respiratory tract of a susceptible host. Invasion aspergillus is rare except in immunocompromised patients, where the infection is characterized by invasion through blood vessel walls that result in tissue infarcts. Aspergillus meningitis is unusual, typically occurring in immunocompromised hosts, and is fatal. Aspergillus tends to be difficult to cultivate in cultures, but the diagnosis can be made by finding septate, acutely branching hyphae in a biopsy specimen. Standard treatment is intravenous amphotericin B; iatraconazole is also used. In general, unless the underlying host defect can be corrected, mortality is high. In this case, there is a moderate amount of leptomeningeal-type enhancement involving the cauda equina. This enhancement pattern is extremely nonspecific and can be seen with pyogenic, fungal, and viral infections.

BIBLIOGRAPHY

Kauffman CA. Opportunistic fungal infections: filamentous fungi and cryptococcosis. *Geriatrics* 1997;52:40–49.
Post MD, Bowen BC, Sze G. Magnetic resonance imaging of spinal infection. *Rheum Dis Clin North Am* 1991;17:773–794.
Post MJD, Sze G, Quencer RM, et al. Gadolinium-enhanced MR in spinal infection. *J Comput Assist Tomogr* 1990;14:721.

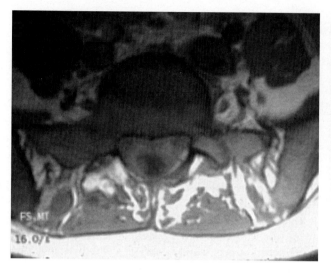

FIGURE 35.1

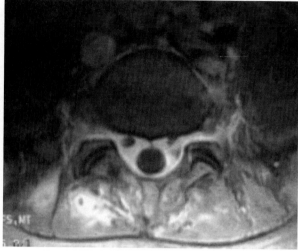

FIGURE 35.2

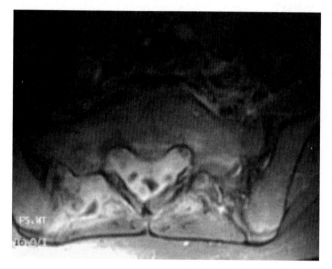

FIGURE 35.3

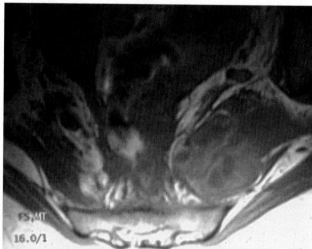

FIGURE 35.4

HISTORY

A 29-year-old with Crohn's disease, fever, and back pain.

FINDINGS

Axial T1-weighted image at the L5–S1 level prior to contrast (Fig. 35.1) shows abnormal diminished signal within the epidural fat in a diffuse fashion, which circumferentially surrounds the exiting roots and thecal sac. Following contrast administration, the T1-weighted image with fat suppression (Fig. 35.2) shows abnormal and diffuse enhancement within the epidural space and surrounding exiting roots. Additional fat-suppressed image through the sacrum (Fig. 35.3) shows abnormal enhancement within the more right dorsal lateral soft tissues with a focal area of low signal consistent with abscess. There is diffuse epidural enhancement, without a focal fluid collection. Axial T1-weighted image without contrast further down within the pelvis (Fig. 35.4) shows a large lobulated mass within the left iliopsoas muscle.

DIAGNOSIS

Epidural phlegmon.

DISCUSSION

The incidence of spinal epidural abscess ranges from 0.2 to 1.96 cases per 10,000, with the higher rates found in more recent literature. This apparent increase may relate to the general aging of the population as well as to the increasing number of spinal procedures and incidents of IV drug abuse. Risk factors for the development of epidural abscess include altered immune status (e.g., diabetes mellitus), renal failure requiring dialysis, alcoholism, and malignancy. Although intravenous drug abuse is a risk factor for epidural abscess, HIV infection does not appear to play a role in the overall increasing incidence of the disease.

Staphylococcus aureus is the organism most commonly associated with epidural abscess, constituting approximately 60% of the cases. It is ubiquitous, tends to form abscesses, and can infect compromised as well as normal hosts. Other gram-positive cocci account for approximately 13% of cases, and gram-negative organisms account for approximately 15%. Most patients are infected by a hematogenous route, with the skin and soft tissues a leading portal. The sites for abscess formation are mainly cervical (25%) and lumbosacral (38%), with half being anterior and a third being circumferential in position. Clinical acute symptomatology classically includes back pain, fever, obtundation, and neurologic deficits. Chronic cases may have less pain and no elevated temperature. The classic course of epidural abscess was described by Rankin and Flothow in four stages; spinal ache, root pain, weakness, paralysis. Acute deterioration from spinal epidural abscess, however, remains unpredictable. Patients may present with abrupt paraplegia and anesthesia. The cause for this precipitous course is unknown, but it is thought to be related to a vascular mechanism (epidural thrombosis and thrombophlebitis, venous infarction).

The primary diagnostic modality in the evaluation of epidural abscess is MR. MR is as sensitive as CT myelography for epidural infection, but it also allows the exclusion of other diagnostic choices, such as herniation, syrinx, tumor, and cord infarction. MR imaging of epidural abscess demonstrates a soft-tissue mass in the epidural space with tapered edges and an associated mass effect on the thecal sac and cord. The epidural masses are usually isointense to the cord on T1-weighted images and of increased signal on T2-weighted images. Occasionally, an epidural mass will be difficult to distinguish when there is associated meningitis (which increases the CSF signal intensity). Post et al. recommended that in these ambiguous cases either CT myelography or perhaps Gd-DTPA enhancement is necessary for full elucidation of the abscess. The patterns of Gd-DTPA enhancement of epidural abscess include (a) diffuse and homogeneous, (b) heterogeneous, and (c) thin peripheral. Post et al. found that Gd-DTPA enhancement was a very useful adjunct for identifying the extent of a lesion when the plain MR scan was equivocal, for demonstrating activity of an infection, and for directing needle biopsy and follow-up treatment. Successful therapy should cause a progressive decrease in enhancement of the paraspinal soft tissues, disk, and vertebral bodies. The role of Gd-DTPA in attempts to distinguish between frank pus and granulation tissue may be clinically significant because there tends to be less surgical enthusiasm for decompression if only phlegmon is shown, versus an abscess collection. Treatment for epidural abscess remains surgical drainage. There is a significant risk to medical management because of its unpredictable clinical course. Despite improvements in imaging and surgical techniques, the mortality rate remains high (23%).

BIBLIOGRAPHY

Hlavin ML, Kaminski HJ, Ross JS, et al. Spinal epidural abscess: a ten-year perspective. *Neurosurgery* 1990;27:177–184.

Post MJD, Quencer RM, Montalvo BM, et al. Spinal infection: evaluation with MR imaging and intraoperative US. *Radiology* 1988;169:765–771.

Post MJD, Sze G, Quencer RM, et al. Gadolinium-enhanced MR in spinal infection. *J Comput Assist Tomogr* 1990;14:721.

Rankin RM, Flothow PG. Pyogenic infection of the spinal epidural space. *West J Surg Obstet Gynecol* 1946;54:320–323.

Sandhu FS, Dillon WP. Spinal epidural abscess: evaluation with contrast-enhanced MR imaging. *Am J Neuroradiol* 1991;12:1087–1093.

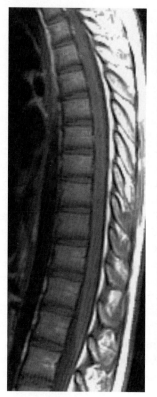 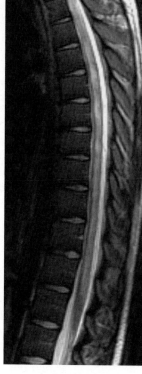 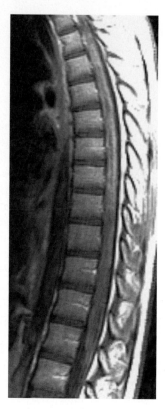

| FIGURE 36.1 | FIGURE 36.2 | FIGURE 36.3 |

HISTORY

A 14-year-old with leg weakness, paresthesias, and ataxia.

FINDINGS

Sagittal T1-weighted image without contrast (Fig. 36.1), sagittal T2-weighted fast spin echo (Fig. 36.2), and sagittal T1-weighted image following contrast administration (Fig. 36.3) show diffuse abnormal increase signal on the T2-weighted image throughout the thoracic cord. There is diffuse and mild enlargement of the thoracic cord as well. Following contrast, there is diffuse enhancement both within the substance of the cord and more linearly along the surface of the cord extending over multiple segments.

DIAGNOSIS

Demyelinating disease (multiple sclerosis).

DISCUSSION

Spinal cord symptoms can be a common presentation of demyelinating disease, particularly multiple sclerosis. Demyelinating plaques in the cervical cord tend to be broad-based along the cord surface or to be seen as well-defined circular areas of demyelination and gliosis within the more central white and gray matter. Lesions show nonspecific signal increase on T2-weighted images and tend to be isointense on T1-weighted images in the relatively acute phase. The cord does not easily display the chronic-phase cavitary lesions that show low signal intensity on T1-weighted images in the brain. More typical late findings in the cord are volume loss with persistent abnormal increase signal on the spin density, short inversion time-recovery (STIR), or T2-weighted images. Following contrast in the acute phase, there is often well-defined enhancement. In this case, there is not only abnormal signal on the T2-weighted image, but gross and diffuse enhancement throughout the thoracic cord. With such diffuse enhancement, the differential would take two pathways—one that the lesion is solely intramedullary and the other that it is a mixture of leptomeningeal enhancement and intramedullary enhancement. For the former, some type of demyelinating disease, whether due to MS or postinfectious myelitis, should be considered. Primary cord tumor would be considered very unlikely due to the overall long segment of distribution. If there is a leptomeningeal and cord pattern, then granulomatous processes such as sarcoidosis would be possible, as well as consideration of leptomeningeal metastatic disease.

BIBLIOGRAPHY

Edwards MK, Farlow MR, Stevens JC. Cranial MR in spinal cord MS: diagnosing patients with isolated spinal cord symptoms. *Am J Neuroradiol* 1986;7:1003–1005.

Filippi M, Yousry TA, Alkadhi H, et al. Spinal cord MRI in multiple sclerosis with multicoil arrays: a comparison between fast spin echo and fast FLAIR. *J Neurol Neurosurg Psychiatry* 1996;61:632–635.

Hittmair K, Mallek R, Prayer D, et al. Spinal cord lesions in patients with multiple sclerosis: comparison of MR pulse sequences. *Am J Neuroradiol* 1996;17:1555–1565.

Marti FJ, Martinez JM, Illa I, et al. Myelopathy of unknown etiology: a clinical follow-up and MRI study of 57 cases. *Acta Neurol Scand* 1989;80:455–460.

Sze G: MR imaging of the spinal cord: Current status and future advances. *Am J Roentgenol* 1992;159:149–159.

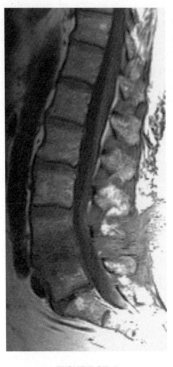

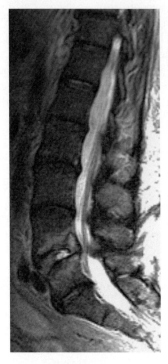

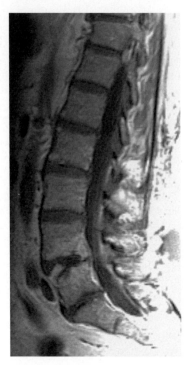

FIGURE 37.1   **FIGURE 37.2**   **FIGURE 37.3**

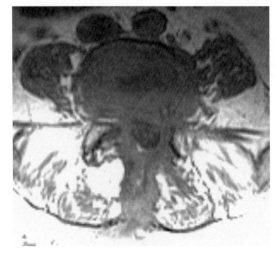

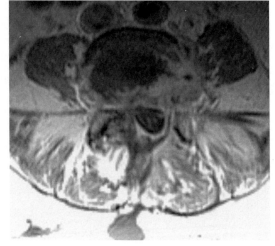

FIGURE 37.4   **FIGURE 37.5**

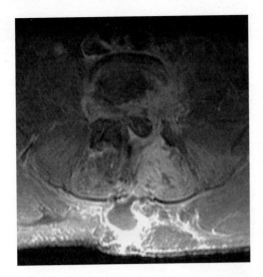

FIGURE 37.6

HISTORY

A 51-year-old with back pain and fever following L4–5 diskectomy.

FINDINGS

Sagittal T1-weighted image without contrast (Fig. 37.1), sagittal T2-weighted fast spin echo image (Fig. 37.2), and sagittal T1-weighted image with contrast (Fig. 37.3) show confluent and abnormal low signal intensity involving the L4–5 vertebral bodies with loss of the distinction of the intervertebral disk. The disk shows abnormal high signal on the T2-weighted image, which extends to the adjacent vertebral bodies. Following contrast, there is irregular and patchy enhancement involving the posterior aspect of the annulus, as well as more anteroinferiorly within the L4–5 annulus. Axial T1-weighted images without contrast (Fig. 37.4), following contrast (Fig. 37.5), and following contrast with fat suppression (Fig. 37.6) show a diffuse abnormal enhancement within the intervertebral disk itself and extending along the left lateral margin of the thecal sac and into the dorsal soft tissue in the midline.

DIAGNOSIS

Postoperative disk space infection.

DISCUSSION

In the postoperative spine, the triad of intervertebral disk space enhancement, annular enhancement, and vertebral body enhancement can lead to the diagnosis of disk space infection, with the appropriate laboratory findings, such as an elevated sedimentation rate. However, normal postoperative patients may also have the triad of annulus enhancement (at the surgical curette site), intervertebral disk enhancement, and vertebral end-plate enhancement without evidence of disk space infection. In these cases, the intervertebral disk enhancement is typically seen as thin bands paralleling the adjacent end plates, and the vertebral body enhancement is presumably the enhancement associated with type I degenerative end-plate changes. Twenty percent of patients may show intervertebral disk enhancement at the surgical level 3 months postoperatively. The enhancing intradiscal tissue most likely reflects granulation or scar tissue related to accelerated disk degeneration postoperatively. This benign degenerative postoperative pattern should be distinguished from the more aggressive amorphous pattern of enhancement seen within the intervertebral disk and annulus with disk space infection.

BIBLIOGRAPHY

Boden SD, Davis DO, Dina TS, et al. Postoperative diskitis: distinguishing early MR imaging findings from normal postoperative disk space changes. *Radiology* 1992;184:765–771.
Ross JS, Zepp R, Modic MT. The postoperative lumbar spine: enhanced MR evaluation of the intervertebral disk. *Am J Neuroradiol* 1996;17:323–331.

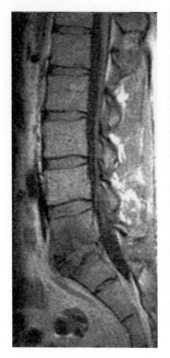 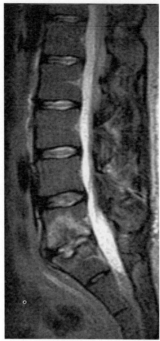 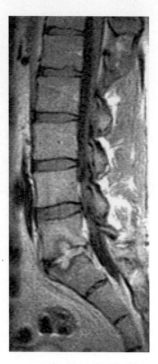

FIGURE 38.1   FIGURE 38.2   FIGURE 38.3

HISTORY

A 44-year-old with back pain and fever.

FINDINGS

Low-field (0.2 Tesla) images. The sagittal T1-weighted image without contrast (Fig. 38.1) show abnormal low signal involving L5–S1 bodies with loss of distinction of the intervertebral disk itself. Sagittal T2-weighted image (Fig. 38.2) shows abnormal high signal within the disk proper at L5–S1, and the high signal within the adjacent L5 and S1 bodies. Sagittal T1-weighted image following contrast (Fig. 38.3) demonstrates diffuse and abnormal enhancement within the vertebral bodies, extending diffusely throughout the intervertebral disk in the areas of end-plate irregularity.

DIAGNOSIS

Disk space infection.

DISCUSSION

MR has been shown to be as accurate and as sensitive as combined bone and gallium scanning and more sensitive than plain films in the evaluation of vertebral osteomyelitis. The MR appearance of pyogenic infection is characteristic, making MR a rapid noninvasive method for the detection of vertebral osteomyelitis and its complications, such as epidural abscess. On T1-weighted images, disk space infection shows confluent decreased signal intensity from the intervertebral disk space and contiguous vertebral bodies relative to the normal vertebral body marrow signal. On T2-weighted images, there is increased signal intensity of these tissues. The intervertebral disk shows abnormal increased signal intensity in a nonanatomic morphology. That is, the intranuclear cleft, a normal anatomic finding in disk in adults over 30 years of age, is absent. The abnormal signal from the end plates may precede the signal changes from the disk itself. MR provides more anatomic detail regarding the adjacent soft tissues and neural elements than radionuclide scanning. Additionally, MR provides a means of differentiating neoplasm and degenerative disease from osteomyelitis. In neoplastic disease, the disk space is almost invariably spared. Degenerative disease tends to show decreased signal from the disk space on T2-weighted images to desiccation of the nucleus. Gallium scanning may be positive earlier than MR in the course of infection. Gallium scanning is probably more sensitive to changes associated with treatment and decreasing inflammation than is MR.

BIBLIOGRAPHY

Modic MT, Steinberg PM, Ross JS, et al. Degenerative disk disease: assessment of changes in vertebral body marrow with MR imaging. *Radiology* 1988;166:193–199.

Post MJD, Sze G, Quencer RM, et al. Gadolinium-enhanced MR in spinal infection. *J Comput Assist Tomogr* 1990;14:721.

Sandhu FS, Dillon WP. Spinal epidural abscess: evaluation with contrast-enhanced MR imaging. *Am J Neuroradiol* 1991;12:1087–1093.

Smith AJ, Weinstein MA, Mizushmia A, et al. MR imaging characteristics of tuberculous spondylitis vs. vertebral osteomyelitis. *Am J Neuroradiol* 1989;10:619.

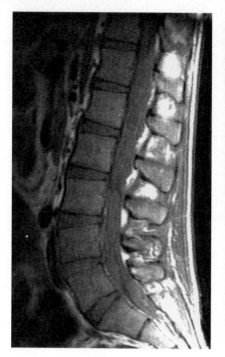

FIGURE 39.1

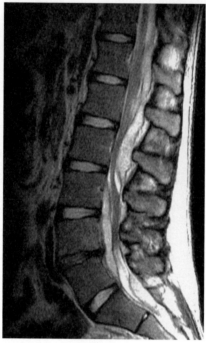

FIGURE 39.2

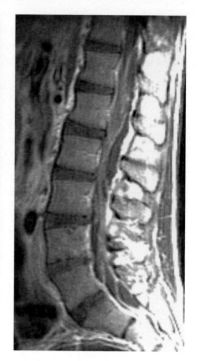

FIGURE 39.3

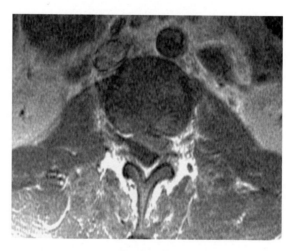

FIGURE 39.4

HISTORY

A 53-year-old with sepsis, and now leg weakness and paresthesias.

FINDINGS

Sagittal T1-weighted image (Fig. 39.1) shows very indistinct thecal sac, which appears to have diffusely increased signal intensity relative to normal CSF signal. No definite vertebral body abnormalities are seen. On the T2-weighted fast spin echo sequence (Fig. 39.2) there is distortion of the roots of the cauda equina, which appear to be displaced anteriorly at the L2–3 level. A heterogeneous mass is located dorsal to the thecal sac spanning the L1 through the S1 levels. This epidural mass is better identified following contrast administration on the sagittal T1-weighted (Fig. 39.3) and axial T1-weighted (Fig. 39.4) images. The epidural mass shows patchy and peripheral enhancement and shows marked displacement of the thecal sac. There is also diffuse and abnormal intradural enhancement along the cauda equina.

DIAGNOSIS

Epidural abscess with meningitis.

DISCUSSION

The incidence of spinal epidural abscess ranges from 0.2 to 1.96 cases per 10,000, with the higher rates found in more recent literature. This apparent increase may relate to the general aging of the population as well as to the increasing number of spinal procedures and incidents of IV drug abuse. Risk factors for the development of epidural abscess include altered immune status (e.g., diabetes mellitus), renal failure requiring dialysis, alcoholism, and malignancy. Although intravenous drug abuse is a risk factor for epidural abscess, HIV infection does not appear to play a role in the overall increasing incidence of the disease. *Staphylococcus aureus* is the organism most commonly associated with epidural abscess, constituting approximately 60% of the cases. It is ubiquitous, tends to form abscesses, and can infect compromised as well as normal hosts. Other gram-positive cocci account for approximately 13% of cases, and gram-negative organisms account for approximately 15%. Most patients are infected by a hematogenous route, with the skin and soft tissues a leading portal. The sites for abscess formation are mainly cervical (25%) and lumbosacral (38%), with half being anterior and a third being circumferential in position. Clinical acute symptomatology classically includes back pain, fever, obtundation, and neurologic deficits. Chronic cases may have less pain and no elevated temperature. Patients may present with abrupt paraplegia and anesthesia. The cause for this precipitous course is unknown, but it is thought to be related to a vascular mechanism (epidural thrombosis and thrombophlebitis, venous infarction).

The primary diagnostic modality in the evaluation of epidural abscess is MR. MR is as sensitive as CT myelography for epidural infection, but it also allows the exclusion of other diagnostic choices such as herniation, syrinx, tumor, and cord infarction. MR imaging of epidural abscess demonstrates a soft-tissue mass in the epidural space with tapered edges and an associated mass effect on the thecal sac and cord. The epidural masses are usually isointense to the cord on T1-weighted images and of increased signal on T2-weighted images. Occasionally, an epidural mass will be difficult to distinguish when there is associated meningitis (which increases the CSF signal intensity). Post et al. recommended that in these ambiguous cases either CT myelography or perhaps Gd-DTPA enhancement is necessary for full elucidation of the abscess. The patterns of Gd-DTPA enhancement of epidural abscess include diffuse and homogeneous, heterogeneous, and thin peripheral. Gd-DTPA enhancement is useful for identifying the extent of a lesion, for demonstrating activity of an infection, and for directing needle biopsy and follow-up treatment. Successful therapy should cause a progressive decrease in enhancement of the paraspinal soft tissues, disk, and vertebral bodies. Treatment for epidural abscess remains immediate surgical drainage.

BIBLIOGRAPHY

Hlavin ML, Kaminski HJ, Ross JS, et al. Spinal epidural abscess: a ten-year perspective. *Neurosurgery* 1990;27:177–184.

Post MJD, Sze G, Quencer RM, et al. Gadolinium-enhanced MR in spinal infection. *J Comput Assist Tomogr* 1990;14:721.

Sandhu FS, Dillon WP. Spinal epidural abscess: evaluation with contrast-enhanced MR imaging. *Am J Neuroradiol* 1991;12:1087–1093.

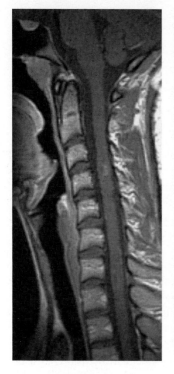

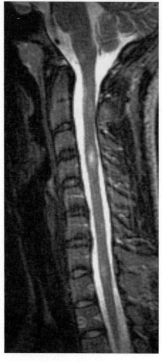

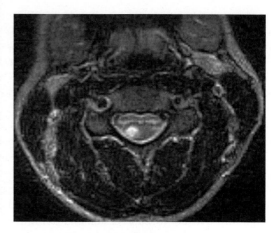

FIGURE 40.1   FIGURE 40.2   FIGURE 40.3

HISTORY

A 33-year-old complaining of right arm clumsiness.

FINDINGS

Sagittal T1-weighted image following contrast (Fig. 40.1) shows that there is mild enhancement of the cord at the C3–4 level. The fast spin echo T2-weighted image (Fig. 40.2) and axial fast spin echo T2 (Fig. 40.3) show focal areas of abnormal increased signal intensity throughout the cervical cord. The T2-weighted sagittal image in particular shows multiple signal abnormalities at the C2, C3–4, C7–T1 levels with mild focal cord enlargement.

DIAGNOSIS

Multiple sclerosis.

DISCUSSION

Multiple sclerosis is usually seen in the second to fifth decades, often manifesting with visual, sensory, and motor dysfunction. Symptoms and signs typically wax and wane. Prevalence of this disorder is higher in northern latitudes and among family members. Histologic sections demon-strate breakdown of myelin sheath, with lymphocytes, plasma cells, and macrophages. The neurons themselves tend to be spared. Spinal cord involvement often presents with weakness and paresthesias of the limbs, Lhermitte's sign, gait disturbance, and disorders of micturition. MR imaging shows linear or elongated increased signal intensity on the T2-weighted spin echo images. These plaques may demonstrate cord enlargement as well as enhancement in more acute episodes. Lesions presenting like this may be indistinguishable from cord neoplasm on one examination, and follow-up is mandatory for the ultimate diagnosis, along with adjunctive studies and imaging of the brain parenchyma.

Cord plaques occur most frequently in the cervical region, and there is a predilection for the posterior aspect (dorsal column) of the cord. The plaques are classically elongated, measure several centimeters in length, and are oriented along the longitudinal axis of the cord. The morphology of the plaques conforms closest to the venous anatomy of the cord rather than to gray/white matter distribution. As in the brain, cord plaques are bright on T2-weighted images and isointense to hypointense on T1-weighted images. Contrast enhancement reflects breakdown in the blood-cord barrier and may be observed in acute lesions with active inflammation or in the margins of activated chronic lesions. Contrast-enhanced MR can therefore be used to measure response to therapy. Initial focal cord swelling or late atrophic changes may be present.

BIBLIOGRAPHY

Edwards MK, Farlow MR, Stevens JC. Cranial MR in spinal cord MS: diagnosing patients with isolated spinal cord symptoms. *Am J Neuroradiol* 1986;7:1003–1005.

Filippi M, Campi A, Martinelli V, et al. Brain and spinal cord MR in benign multiple sclerosis: a follow-up study. *J Neurol Sci* 1996;143:143–149.

Keiper MD, Grossman RI, Brunson JC, et al. The low sensitivity of fluid-attenuated inversion-recovery MR in the detection of multiple sclerosis of the spinal cord. *Am J Neuroradiol* 1997;18:1035–1039.

Mascalchi M, Dal PG, Bartolozzi C. Effectiveness of the short TI inversion recovery (STIR) sequence in MR imaging of intramedullary spinal lesions. *Magn Reson Imaging* 1993;11:17–25.

Miller DH, Grossman RI, Reingold SC, et al. The role of magnetic resonance techniques in understanding and managing multiple sclerosis. *Brain* 1998;121:3–24.

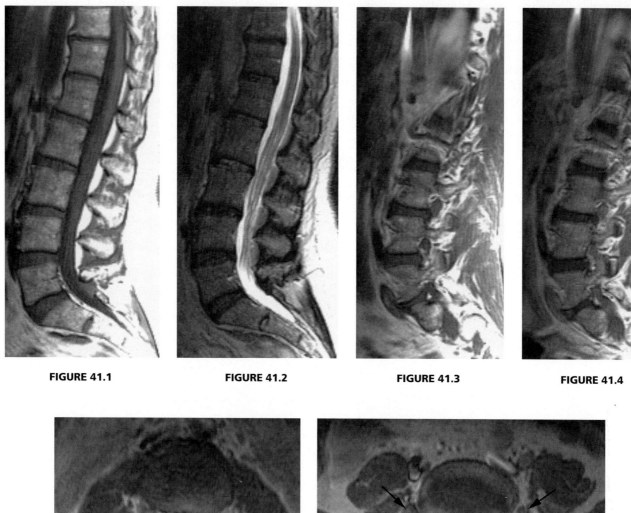

FIGURE 41.1   **FIGURE 41.2**   **FIGURE 41.3**   **FIGURE 41.4**

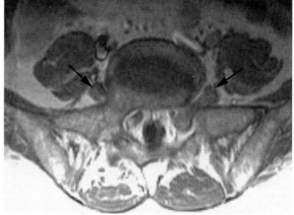

FIGURE 41.5   **FIGURE 41.6**

HISTORY

A 53-year-old with leg weakness and EMG showing chronic sensorimotor polyneuropathy.

FINDINGS

Midline sagittal T1-weighted (Fig. 41.1) and fast spin echo sagittal T2-weighted (Fig. 41.2) images show enlargement and thickening of the roots of the cauda equina in a diffuse fashion. There is no evidence of significant extradural disease. Parasagittal T1-weighted image prior to contrast (Fig. 41.3), and following contrast (Fig. 41.4) show diffuse enlargement of the exiting roots, including the nerve root ganglion with mild diffuse enhancement. Axial T1-weighted images at the L3–4 level (Fig. 41.5) and at the L5–S1 level (Fig. 41.6) also show diffuse enlargement of the peripheral nerves (*arrows*).

DIAGNOSIS

Hereditary motor and sensory neuropathy (Charcot-Marie-Tooth disease).

DISCUSSION

Hereditary diseases of peripheral nerves have been classified by many different criteria throughout the years. The initial classification was clinical, moved on to histopathology, then involved the pattern of inheritance. Nerve conduction velocity became a major feature determining classification; it has now been superseded by molecular biology, which allows identification of the affected gene products. Numerically, the most important group is Charcot-Marie-Tooth (CMT) disease or peroneal muscular atrophy. The term *hereditary motor and sensory neuropathy* (HSMN) has also been used as a formal designation. This group accounts for 90% of all hereditary neuropathies, and the prevalence in the United States is about 40 per 100,000 people (more common than myasthenia gravis and twice as common as Duchenne dystrophy). The most common forms are type 1, with autosomal dominant inheritance, demyelinating neuropathy with slow conduction velocities, and histologic evidence of demyelination with remyelination in the form of "onion bulb" formations. Type 2 is clinically similar, including sensory loss, but conductions are normal, and there is no histologic evidence of demyelination. The inheritance pattern is variable. The most severe form is autosomal recessive type 3, with an onset in early childhood, and extreme disability from a hypertrophic demyelinating disorder. In types 1 and 2, symptoms generally begin in childhood or adolescence. The first signs may be skeletal, with pes cavus or other deformity of the feet, or scoliosis. Disproportionate thinness of the lower legs can be evident before there is a gait disorder with footdrop. The weakness and wasting are usually symmetric, and progression is slow. Ultimately, the hands are also affected, and that may be more disabling than the gait disorder. Cranial nerves are generally spared.

There is no specific drug or gene therapy for these diseases. Treatment is directed to mechanical assistance for leg weakness, surgical correction of deformities, and physical therapy. The time course of types 1 or 2 is so slow that most people enjoy a productive life. Children with the Dejerine-Sottas form, however, have serious problems and may never walk.

The MR imaging examination of the lumbar spine may show diffusely enlarged cauda equina, nerve roots, and ganglia. With the appropriate family history and clinical presentation, the findings of diffusely enlarged nerve roots support the diagnosis of hereditary motor and sensory neuropathy, type I (Charcot-Marie-Tooth). In severe cases the hypertrophic nerve roots may require multilevel decompressive laminectomy to relieve myelopathy, spinal claudication, or radiculopathy.

BIBLIOGRAPHY

Choi SK, Bowers RP, Buckthal PE. MR imaging in hypertrophic neuropathy: a case of hereditary motor and sensory neuropathy, type I (Charcot-Marie-Tooth). *Clin Imaging* 1990;14:204–207.

Lovelace RE, Rowland LP. Hereditary neuropathies. In: Rowland LP, ed. *Merritts textbook of neurology*, 9th ed. New York: Williams & Wilkins, 1995;652–655.

Rosen SA, Wang H, Cornblath DR, et al. Compression syndromes due to hypertrophic nerve roots in hereditary motor sensory neuropathy type I. *Neurology* 1989;39:1173–1177.

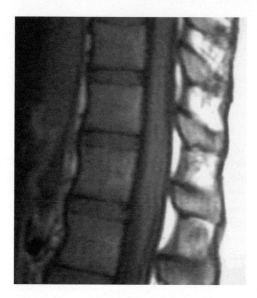

FIGURE 42.1

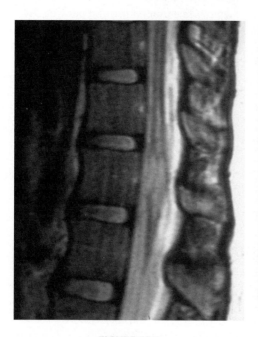

FIGURE 42.2

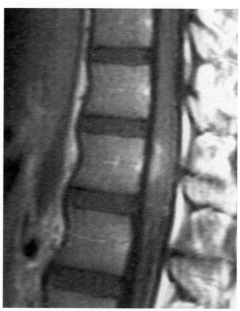

FIGURE 42.3

HISTORY

A 38-year-old with new onset of leg weakness.

FINDINGS

Sagittal T1-weighted image before contrast (Fig. 42.1) shows mild and diffuse enlargement of the conus. No focal signal abnormalities otherwise are identified. The fast spin echo sagittal T2-weighted image (Fig. 42.2) shows high signal intensity involving the conus both centrally and extending to the surface. This extends over approximately one and one-half vertebral body segments. Following contrast administration, the sagittal T1-weighted image (Fig. 42.3) shows irregular and ill-defined enhancement involving the substance of the conus but extending to the periphery of the distal cord.

DIAGNOSIS

Postinfectious myelitis involving conus.

DISCUSSION

A variety of viruses and bacteria can give rise to postinfectious myelitis, or the clinical syndrome of "transverse myelitis." These are generally thought to reflect an immunologic response against the central nervous system as a final common etiology. Pathologically, the lesions are confined to the white matter showing patchy myelin breakdown as well as perivenous lymphocytic infiltration with occasional plasma cells. The neurons themselves are normal. Various agents have been implicated, such as smallpox, chicken pox, measles and German measles, mumps, influenza, herpes simplex, and Epstein-Barr virus. Bacterial infections such as scarlet fever, pertussis, and mycoplasma may also present with transverse myelitis.

Clinically, their symptoms include leg weakness, sensory disturbance in the legs, back pain, and radicular pain. Clinical symptoms usually evolve rapidly from the time of onset. Respiratory insufficiency can be present in those with high thoracic or cervical levels of involvement. Recovery tends to begin 2 to 12 weeks after onset and may continue for years. A good recovery with no residual deficits can be expected in about one-third of these patients. Imaging of acute transverse myelitis has shown cord enlargement and increased signal on T2-weighted sequences in the acute phase. These findings may also be seen in the acute phase of multiple sclerosis. Tumor is also a diagnostic consideration, but clinical onset and course usually allow distinction.

BIBLIOGRAPHY

Ford B, Tampieri D, Francis G. Long-term follow-up of acute partial transverse myelopathy. *Neurology* 1992;42:250–252.
Holtas S, Basibuyuk N, Fredriksson K. MRI in acute transverse myelopathy. *Neuroradiology* 1993;35:221–226.
Thorpe JW, Kidd D, Moseley IF, et al. Spinal MRI in patients with suspected multiple sclerosis and negative brain MRI. *Brain* 1996;119:709–714.

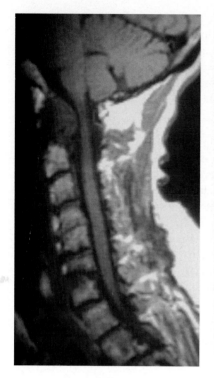

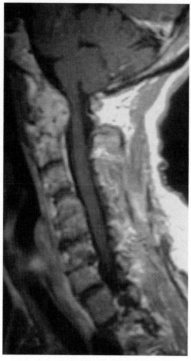

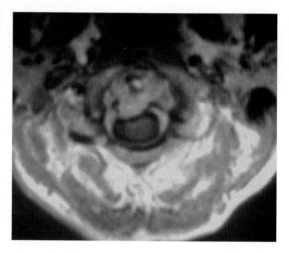

FIGURE 43.1   **FIGURE 43.2**   **FIGURE 43.3**

HISTORY

A 66-year-old with arm and leg weakness.

FINDINGS

Sagittal T1-weighted image without contrast (Fig. 43.1), sagittal T1-weighted image, and axial T1-weighted images with contrast (Figs. 43.2 and 42.3) demonstrate a large soft-tissue mass involving the dontoid process with extension into the epidural space at the cranial cervical junction. This appears separate from the anterior arch of C1. There is diffuse but somewhat heterogeneous enhancement of the lesion. There is evidence of loss of disk space height at several levels in the cervical spine with several small areas of end-plate irregularity.

DIAGNOSIS

Rheumatoid arthritis

DISCUSSION

Involvement of the cervical spine occurs in 36% to 88% of patients affected with rheumatoid arthritis. Several different types of subluxations occur, including (a) anterior atlantoaxial, (b) vertical subluxation of the odontoid, (c) posterior atlantoaxial (associated with an eroded odontoid), (d) lateral subluxation of C1, (e) subaxial subluxation. With anterior atlantoaxial subluxation, clinical manifestations include occipital temporal and retroorbital pain. Myelopathy results from cord compression between the odontoid and the anteriorly displaced posterior arch of C1. The atlantodental interval is measured in flexion on lateral views and should not be greater than 2.5 to 3 mm in adults. Vertical subluxation of the odontoid into the foramen magnum may compress the cervicomedullary junction, leading to myelopathy or death. On the lateral plain film, using the Redlund-Johnell method (which evaluates the distance between the base of C2 and McGregor's line), the normal values are 34 mm or greater in men and 28 mm or greater in women. Likewise, the upper cervical cord is often found to be compressed in patients with a subarachnoid space of 13 mm or less.

Following surgery, studies have described decreased size of the periodontoid pannus in patients with atlantoaxial subluxation. It is assumed that the pannus reduction is a result of the atlantoaxial immobility from surgery. Likewise, some authors have concluded that posterior fixation by itself may lead to sufficient decompression by resolving the periodontol pannus and that anterior approaches for decompression may not be as necessary.

BIBLIOGRAPHY

Bell GR, Stearns KL. Flexion-extension MRI of the upper rheumatoid cervical spine. *Orthopedics* 1991;14:969–974.

Bundschuh C, Modic MT, Kearney F, et al. Rheumatoid arthritis of the cervical spine: surface-coil MR imaging. *Am J Neuroradiol* 1988;9:565–571.

Dvorak J, Grob D, Baumgartner H, et al. Functional evaluation of the spinal cord by magnetic resonance imaging in patients with rheumatoid arthritis and instability of upper cervical spine. *Spine* 1989;14:1057–1064.

Komusi T, Munro T, Harth M. Radiologic review: the rheumatoid cervical spine. *Semin Arthritis Rheum* 1985;14:187–195.

Lipson SJ. Rheumatoid arthritis in the cervical spine. *Clin Orthop Relat Res* 1989;239:121–127.

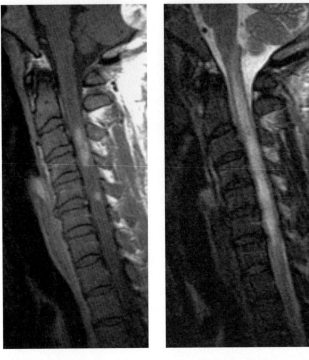

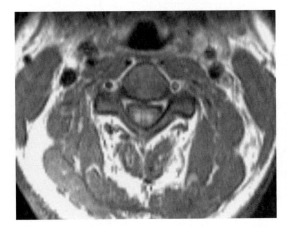

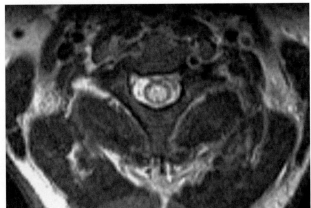

| FIGURE 44.1 | FIGURE 44.2 |

| FIGURE 44.3 | FIGURE 44.4 |

HISTORY

A 39-year-old with gradual-onset myelopathy.

FINDINGS

Sagittal T1-weighted image after contrast administration (Fig. 44.1) shows scattered areas of fairly well-defined enhancement within the cervical cord at the C3–4 and C5–6

levels. The sagittal T2-weighted fast spin echo sequence (Fig. 44.2) shows diffuse abnormal increase signal intensity within the cervical cord spanning the C1 through C6–7 levels. Axial T1-weighted image following contrast administration (Fig. 44.3) again demonstrates the central enhancement within the cord. Axial fast spin echo T2-weighted sequence (Fig. 44.4) confirms the predominantly central area of high signal intensity with relative sparing of the periphery of the cord.

DIAGNOSIS

Sarcoidosis.

DISCUSSION

Sarcoidosis is a multisystem granulomatous disease of unknown cause. It is diagnosed by noncaseating granulomas, with supportive laboratory and imaging findings. These include primarily chest radiographs and angiotensin-converting enzyme (ACE) levels. The true positive yield from ACE is 75%. Areas of involvement are most commonly the lung and hila, with eye and skin involvement next common. The CNS is affected in up to 5% of cases. Areas of CNS involvement include the cranial nerves (cranial polyneuritis), basal cisterns (meningitis with hydrocephalus), and hypothalamus (diabetes insipidus). Other clinical syndromes include a peripheral neuropathy and myopathy. Approximately 69 cases of spinal cord involvement are reported in the literature. Pathologic changes include sarcoid tissue in the meninges and parenchyma, with areas of infarction resulting from occlusion of small vessels by the granulomas.

MR shows direct cord involvement (increased cord size) and increased signal on T2-weighted images, combined with evidence of leptomeningeal enhancement. Patchy multifocal enhancement of the cord (which is broad-based) and adjacent to the cord surface is typical.

BIBLIOGRAPHY

Atkinson R, Ghelman B, Tsairis P, et al. Sarcoidosis presenting as cervical radiculopathy: a case report and literature review. *Spine* 1982;7:412–416.

Lexa FJ, Grossman RI. MR of sarcoidosis in the head and spine: spectrum of manifestations and radiographic response to steroid therapy. *Am J Neuroradiol* 1994;15:973–982.

Miller DH, Kendall BE, Barter S, et al. Magnetic resonance imaging in central nervous system sarcoidosis. *Neurology* 1988;38:378–383.

Pascuzzi RM, Shapiro SA, Rau AN, et al. Sarcoid myelopathy. *J Neuroimaging* 1996;6:61–62.

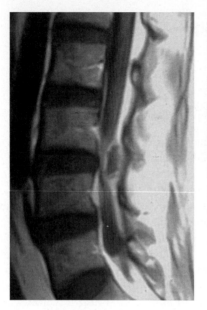 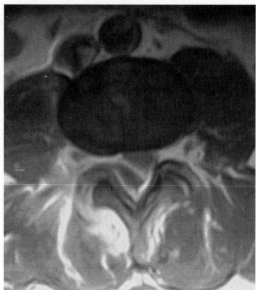

FIGURE 45.1   **FIGURE 45.2**

HISTORY

A 37-year-old with new-onset right back pain.

FINDINGS

Sagittal and axial T1-weighted images following contrast administration (Figs. 45.1 and 45.2) demonstrate a focal area of central low signal intensity adjacent to the right L3–4 facet that extends into the dorsal epidural space. The mass shows peripheral enhancement and effaces the dorsal aspect of the thecal sac. There is no abnormality involving the vertebral bodies or intervertebral disks. The intradural contents are otherwise normal in appearance. There is moderate but ill-defined enhancement involving the right facet joint and extending into the adjacent soft tissue and dorsal musculature.

DIAGNOSIS

Septic facet joint.

DISCUSSION

Before the advent of antibiotic therapy, spinal osteomyelitis epidural abscess was often an acute virulent disease that caused death from septic complications. Patients who survived long enough to develop abscesses were generally treated by abscess drainage and immobilization. Since antibiotic therapy has become all-pervasive, the disease has become more insidious. Dilemmas may arise because clinical and laboratory findings mimic a neoplastic, traumatic, or inflammatory condition. Reliance on conventional radiographs can allow extensive bony destruction to take place before therapy is instituted. The sources for bacteremia that seed osteomyelitis or a septic facet are generally genitourinary, dermal, and respiratory.

Infection may not be considered in the differential for back pain because it remains an uncommon disorder (less than 1% of all cases of osteomyelitis). Once infection is considered, accurate imaging is necessary to provide invasive tests for a microbiologic diagnosis or surgical drainage. Because abnormalities that appear on plain radiographs usually take days to weeks to become manifest, radionuclide studies have been the primary imaging modality for vertebral osteomyelitis.

Radionuclides most commonly used for detecting inflammatory changes of the spine are technetium 99m (99mTc) phosphate complexes, gallium (67Ga) citrate, and indium-111-labeled white blood cells. Although scintigraphy with 99mTc and 67Ga compounds is sensitive to infection, it is also nonspecific. Healing fractures, sterile inflammatory reactions, tumors, and loosened prosthetic devices can show increased uptake. Indium-111 has several advantages compared with other radionuclides, including higher target-to-background ratios, better image quality, and more intense uptake by abscesses. Its main disadvantage is its accumulation within any inflammatory lesion, whether infectious or not. The radionuclide study also takes time to perform—hours to days. Computed tomography has played a minor role in cases with bony or soft-tissue components and is not considered a mainstay for the diagnosis of disk space infection. Literature comparing MR with the more conventional modalities in diagnosing inflammatory processes continues to grow. In appropriate situations MR appears to have a sensitivity for detecting vertebral osteomyelitis that exceeds that of plain films and CT and approaches or equals that of radionuclide studies. In this case, the surrounding soft-tissue enhancement with irregular margins leads to the diagnosis of infection. The differential diagnoses would include a large joint effusion secondary to degenerative disease, or a large synovial cyst.

BIBLIOGRAPHY

Ergan M, Macro M, Benhamou CL, et al. Septic arthritis of lumbar facet joints: a review of six cases. *Rev Rhum Engl Ed* 1997;64:386–395.

Fujiwara A, Tamai K, Yamato M, et al. Septic arthritis of a lumbar facet joint: report of a case with early MRI findings. *J Spinal Disord* 1998;11:452–453.

Heenan SD, Britton J. Septic arthritis in a lumbar facet joint: a rare cause of an epidural abscess. *Neuroradiology* 1995;37:462–464.

Rousselin B, Gires F, Vallee C, et al. Case report 627: septic arthritis of lumbar facet joint as initial manifestation of spondylodiscitis. *Skeletal Radiol* 1990;19:453–455.

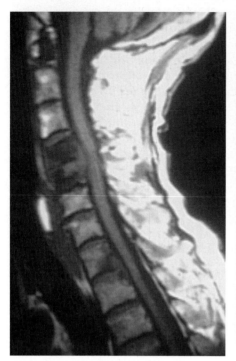

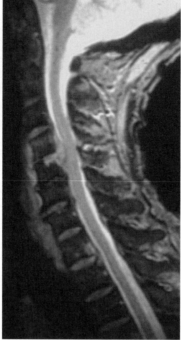

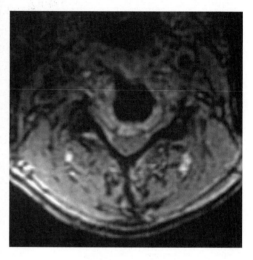

FIGURE 46.1   FIGURE 46.2   FIGURE 46.3

HISTORY

A 46-year-old with gradual-onset neck pain.

FINDINGS

Sagittal T1-weighted (Fig 46.1), sagittal T2-weighted (Fig 46.2), and axial gradient echo image (Fig 46.3) show multiple focal abnormalities. Specifically, there is abnormally low signal involving the C4–5 vertebral bodies and adjacent disk, and more posteriorly within the T1 and T2 bodies. There is epidural extension of soft tissue at the C4–5 level with moderate effacement of anterior thecal sac and mild effacement of the cord. There is relative preservation of the disk space at the T1–2 level but involvement at the C5–6 level.

DIAGNOSIS

Tuberculous osteomyelitis/spondylitis.

DISCUSSION

Tuberculous spondylitis has been noted to demonstrate findings more typical of neoplasms than of pyogenic spondylitis. These findings include sparing of the intervertebral disk space, with no abnormal increased signal on T2-weighted images; preferential involvement of the posterior elements and posterior portions of the vertebral bodies; involvement of more than two vertebral bodies; and large paraspinal soft-tissue masses. Tuberculous spondylitis begins in the anterior-inferior portion of the vertebral body, with spread beneath the longitudinal ligaments. The intervertebral disk is commonly not involved. The lack of proteolytic enzymes in mycobacteria has been touted as the cause of intervertebral disk space preservation. With the predilection for multiple vertebral body and posterior element involvement, the distinction from metastatic disease may be impossible, except when correlated with history. In North America spinal tuberculosis is most common in young adults (30 to 45 years) and has an insidious onset (months to years). Also to be included in the differential diagnosis are other unusual infections, such as actinomycosis (which can also spread by subligamentous route) and hydatid disease (which can produce vertebral body destruction and a paraspinal mass). Similarly, type I vertebral body changes should be considered, because both type I changes and spinal tuberculosis can show increased signal on T1-weighted images from adjacent vertebral bodies and a narrowed disk space without increased signal on T2-weighted images.

BIBLIOGRAPHY

Del COJ, Gower DJ, McWhorter JM. Changing concepts in spinal epidural abscess: a report of 29 cases. *Neurosurgery* 1990;27:185–192.

Post MJD, Sze G, Quencer RM, et al. Gadolinium-enhanced MR in spinal infection. *J Comput Assist Tomogr* 1990;14(5):721–729.

Sharif HS, Aideyan OA, Clark DC, et al. Brucellar and tuberculous spondylitis: comparative imaging features. *Radiology* 1989;171:419–425.

Smith AS, Weinstein MA, Mizushima A, et al. MR imaging characteristics of tuberculous spondylitis vs vertebral osteomyelitis. *Am J Roentgenol* 1989;153:399–405.

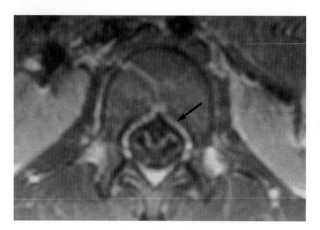

FIGURE 47.1

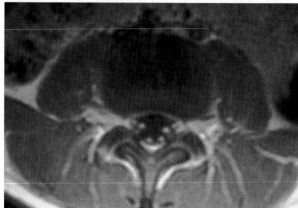

FIGURE 47.2

HISTORY

A 25-year-old with progressing leg weakness.

FINDINGS

Two axial T1-weighted images (Figs. 47.1 and 47.2) following contrast administration demonstrate marked enhancement of several nerve roots of the cauda equina but particularly involving the ventral roots (*arrow*). No discrete mass is identified otherwise. Vertebral bodies and posterior elements in the adjacent soft tissues are normal. Images courtesy of R. Murray, Rockford, Ill.

DIAGNOSIS

Guillain-Barré syndrome.

DISCUSSION

The Guillain-Barré syndrome or acute inflammatory demyelinating neuropathy is characterized by acute onset of peripheral and cranial nerve dysfunction. The cause of the Guillain-Barré syndrome is unknown but is thought to be immune mediated. Clinical findings include an ascending progressive muscle weakness that is more prominent proximally, areflexia, a mild distal sensory loss, and bilateral facial weakness. Autonomic dysfunction may occur, causing fluctuations in blood pressure, temperature, and heart rate. Rarely, patients may die, particularly where autonomic dysfunction and arrhythmias are prominent. The condition worsens for several days to 3 weeks, followed by a period of stability, and then gradual improvement to normal or nearly normal function. CSF protein may be normal during the initial stage of the illness but usually rises within a few days. Nerve conduction studies are abnormal early in the course of the disease. Early plasmapheresis or intravenous infusion of human gamma globulins accelerates recovery and diminishes the incidence of long-term disability. Up to 90% of patients make a complete recovery. Histologically, the syndrome shows focal segmental demyelination with perivascular lymphocytes and monocyte infiltrates. Contrast enhancement of lumbosacral roots in patients with chronic inflammatory demyelinating polyradiculoneuropathy and Guillain-Barré syndrome has been described, but not in association with other demyelinating neuropathies. The clinical history and imaging findings will be quite specific for Guillain-Barré, particularly if there is isolated ventral nerve enhancement. If the clinical history is lacking, then the imaging findings are quite nonspecific and other possibilities would include viral or bacterial meningitis, leptomeningeal metastasis, and granulomatous disease.

BIBLIOGRAPHY

Bertorini T, Halford H, Lawrence J, et al. Contrast-enhanced magnetic resonance imaging of the lumbosacral roots in the dysimmune inflammatory polyneuropathies *J Neuroimaging* 1995;5:9–15.

Byun WM, Park WK, Park BH, et al. Guillain-Barré syndrome: MR imaging findings of the spine in eight patients. *Radiology* 1998;208:137–141.

Fuchigami T, Iwata F, Noguchi Y, et al. Magnetic resonance imaging of the cauda equina in two patients with Guillain-Barré syndrome. *Acta Paediatr Jpn* 1997;39:607–610.

Gorson KC, Ropper AH, Muriello MA, et al. Prospective evaluation of MRI lumbosacral nerve root enhancement in acute Guillain-Barré syndrome. *Neurology* 1996;47:813–817.

Iwata F, Utsumi Y. MR imaging in Guillain-Barré syndrome. *Pediatr Radiol* 1997;27:36–38.

Rowland LP. *Merritt's textbook of neurology,* 9th ed. Baltimore: Williams & Wilkins, 1995.

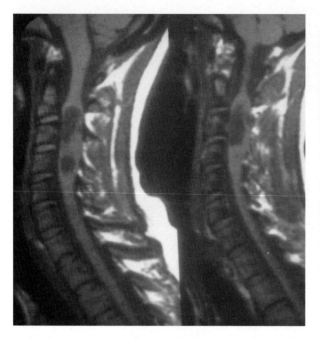

FIGURE 48.1

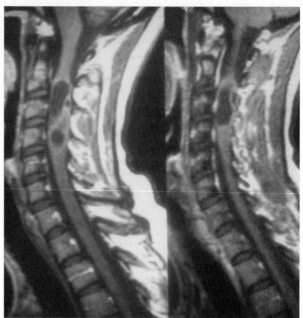

FIGURE 48.2

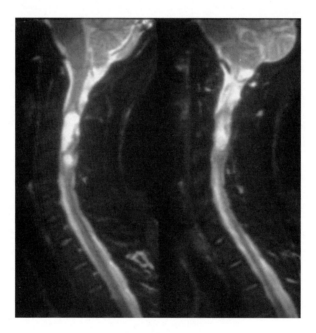

FIGURE 48.3

HISTORY

A 33-year-old with myelopathy.

FINDINGS

Pairs of sagittal T1-weighted images without contrast (Fig. 48.1), T1-weighted images following contrast material (Fig. 48.2), and sagittal T2-weighted images (Fig. 48.3) demonstrate a complex cystic and solid mass involving the upper cervical cord, with fusiform cord enlargement. There is mild and patchy enhancement following contrast administration. Overall degree of enhancement is small given the overall size and complexity of the lesion. The lesion does appear to fusiformly enlarge the cord and appears intramedullary. Images courtesy of Renato Mendoca, M.D. Sao Paulo, Brazil.

DIAGNOSIS

Spinal cysticercosis.

DISCUSSION

Cysticercosis is the most common CNS parasitic disease worldwide, being endemic in many areas, such as Mexico, Central and South America, Asia, India, and Africa. The infection arises through ingesting the eggs of the pork tapeworm (*Taenia solium*), usually in contaminated food or water. The egg shell then degenerates in the intestinal tract, the embryos invade the vessels of the intestinal tract and are disseminated hematogenously to the brain, skeletal muscle, and other tissues before developing into larvae after approximately 2 months. The central nervous system is involved in 60% to 90% of patients with cysticercosis. Spinal cysticercosis is relatively rare and may involve the subarachnoid space, the cord, or the epidural space. Intramedullary cysticercosis can be manifest as round cysts with eccentric nodules (scolex) and ring shape enhancement. Edema and enlargement of the cord can occur. Subarachnoid involvement can be a cystic mass compressing the cord and nerve roots, with minimal enhancement. Multiseptated cysts can also occur with leptomeningeal enhancement. In intramedullary disease, as in this case, there is fusiform enlargement in multicystic areas with very minimal enhancement. In North America, most commonly this pattern would reflect an astrocytoma. However, with appropriate clinical history of travel into endemic areas, more unusual disease, such as neurocysticercosis, may be contemplated.

BIBLIOGRAPHY

Carpio A, Escobar A, Hauser WA. Cysticercosis and epilepsy: a critical review. *Epilepsia* 1998;39:1025–1040.
Chang KH, Han MH. MRI of CNS parasitic diseases. *J Magn Reson Imaging* 1998;8:297–307.
Garg RK. Neurocysticercosis. *Postgrad Med J* 1998;74:321–326.
Garg RK, Nag D. Intramedullary spinal cysticercosis: response to albendazole: case reports and review of literature. *Spinal Cord* 1998;36:67–70.
Mohanty A. Spinal Intramedullary cysticercosis. *Neurosurgery* 1997;40(1):82–87.

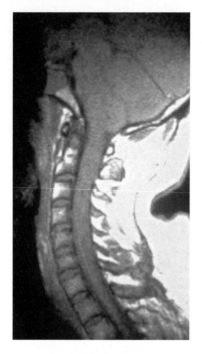

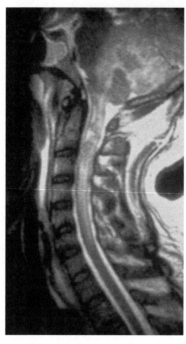

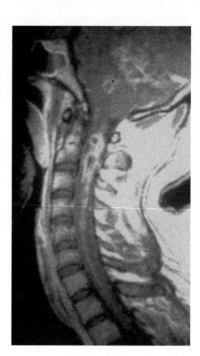

| FIGURE 49.1 | FIGURE 49.2 | FIGURE 49.3 |

HISTORY

A 37-year-old with leg and arm weakness, fever, and obtundation.

FINDINGS

Sagittal T1-weighted image prior to contrast (Fig. 49.1), sagittal T2-weighted image (Fig. 49.2), and sagittal T1-weighted image following contrast administration (Fig. 49.3) show marked enlargement of the upper cervical cord with diffuse and heterogeneous increase signal on the T2-weighted images. The abnormal signal extends throughout the dorsal brain stem and cerebellar hemispheres and vermis. Multiple areas of ring enhancement as well as additional, more solid and irregular areas of enhancement are seen within the posterior fossa and the upper cervical cord. There is a gas-fluid level within the sphenoid sinus. Images courtesy of Joseph Illes, M.D., Johannesburg, South Africa.

DIAGNOSIS

Intramedullary abscess.

DISCUSSION

The most typical infection involving the cervical spine would be considered osteomyelitis-diskitis and epidural abscess. In this case, the abnormality is clearly intramedullary and shows a large area of irregular ring enhancement involving the posterior fossa and extending into the upper cervical cord. The primary differential would be a posterior fossa tumor that spread to the upper cervical cord. In this case, this is all secondary to abscess, which has extended from the posterior fossa into the cervical cord due to *Streptococcus faecalis*. *Staphylococcus aureus* is the most common offending bacterial organism associated with osteomyelitis/diskitis and a cord abscess as well. If the patient is immunocompromised, then *S. aureus* is still going to be the most likely organism but would include other, more unusual lesions such as gram-negative bacteria and *Nocardia*. Cord abscess is a very rare lesion compared with the much more common osteomyelitis/diskitis and epidural abscess.

BIBLIOGRAPHY

Chan CT, Gold WL. Intramedullary abscess of the spinal cord in the antibiotic era: clinical features, microbial etiologies, trends in pathogenesis, and outcomes. *Clin Infect Dis* 1998;27:619–626.

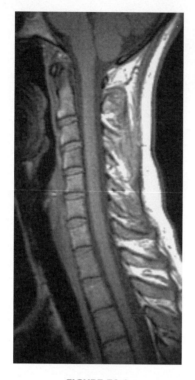

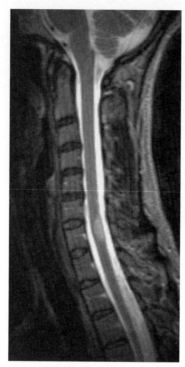

FIGURE 50.1

FIGURE 50.2

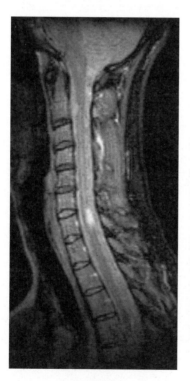

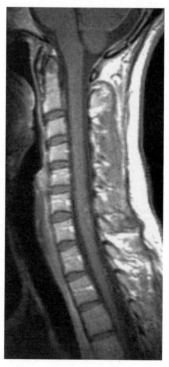

FIGURE 50.3

FIGURE 50.4

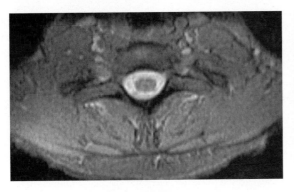

FIGURE 50.5

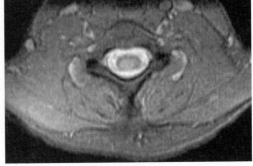

FIGURE 50.6

HISTORY

A 28-year-old with optic neuritis.

FINDINGS

Sagittal T1-weighted image without contrast (Fig. 50.1), sagittal fast spin echo T2-weighted image (Fig. 50.2), fast spin echo short inversion time inversion-recovery (STIR) (Fig. 50.3) demonstrate a focal area of abnormal signal within the cervical cord at the C6–7 level. There is mild enlargement of the cord. Following contrast administration is a very mild enhancement involving the dorsal aspect of the cord (Fig. 50.4). Axial three-dimensional gradient echo sequence at the normal cord level at C7–T1 (Fig. 50.5) should be contrasted against the abnormal cord at the C6–7 level (Fig. 50.6), which shows high signal centrally and dorsally contrasted with the normal-appearing lower signal intensity around the periphery.

DIAGNOSIS

Multiple sclerosis.

DISCUSSION

Fast spin echo (FSE) is the gold standard for spinal sagittal T2 and spin density weighted imaging. In conventional spin echo techniques, one Ky line (phase encode) is obtained for each 90- to 180-degree pulse pair. A 256 × 256 matrix would require 256 such pulses. FSE techniques are based on a modification of the original rapid acquisition relaxation enhancement (RARE) techniques, where all the Ky lines were acquired after one 90-degree pulse, with the number of 180-degree pulses equal to the total number of Ky lines. If some portions (or segment) of all the Ky lines are obtained after a 90 pulse using multiple 180-degree pulses, then the sequence is hybrid RARE, also called FSE, or turbo spin echo (SE). In routine SE imaging, the image contrast is controlled by the TR and the TE. New parameters were added with FSE, such as echo train length and echo spacing, that can be manipulated to alter image contrast. New artifacts and appearances are also added by these techniques, such as T2 filtering (imaging blurring), bright fat, and diminished sensitivity to susceptibility effects. Since multiple echos are obtained at different echo times (TEs) in the FSE sequence, the overall image has not one true TE but an effective TE.

STIR has shown a high sensitivity for musculoskeletal pathology due to the synergistic effects of prolonged T1 and T2 in abnormal tissues, coupled with the improved contrast/noise with fat suppression. STIR has been favorably compared with T1- and T2-weighted FSE, conventional spin echo (CSE), and fat sat FSE in the detection of vertebral metastatic disease.

The use of fast STIR for intramedullary disease is less well known. In the analysis by Hittmair et al., the fast STIR sequence was best for detecting multiple sclerosis lesions and showed lesions that were missed on other, more routine techniques, such as FSE. Their technique included asymmetric sampling with one echo collected before the TE effective and six echo collected after (echo train of 8), six averages, and a cephalocaudal phase encode direction. The cephalocaudal phase encode direction is typical for FSE sagittal spine sequences. The fast STIR will require a slighter short TI and more signal averages than the conventional STIR sequence due to the contribution of stimulated echos. The overall image quality tends to be rather noisy, but the utility is provided by the high contrast to noise. This technique appears very useful for cervical cord disease but is more prone to motion artifact and suffers in the evaluation of thoracic cord disease.

BIBLIOGRAPHY

Baker LL, Goodman SB, Perkash I, et al. Benign versus pathologic compression fractures of vertebral bodies: assessment with conventional spin-echo, chemical-shift, and STIR MR imaging. *Radiology* 1990;174:495–502.

Dwyer AJ, Frank JA, Sank VJ, et al. Short-Ti inversion-recovery pulse sequence: analysis and initial experience in cancer imaging. *Radiology* 1988;168:827–836.

Georgy BA, Hesselink JR. MR imaging of the spine: recent advances in pulse sequences and special techniques. *Am J Roentgenol* 1994;162:923–934.

Hilfiker P, Zanetti M, Debatin JF, et al. Fast spin-echo inversion-recovery imaging versus fast T2-weighted spin- echo imaging in bone marrow abnormalities. *Invest Radiol* 1995;30:110–114.

Hittmair K, Trattnig S, Herold CJ, et al. Comparison between conventional and fast spin-echo stir sequences. *Acta Radiol* 1996;37:943–949.

Jones KM, Mulkern RV, Schwartz RB, et al. Fast spin-echo MR imaging of the brain and spine: current concepts. *Am J Roentgenol* 1992;158:1313–1320.

Mehta RC, Marks MP, Hinks RS, et al. MR evaluation of vertebral metastases: T1-weighted, short-inversion–time inversion recovery, fast spin-echo, and inversion-recovery fast spin-echo sequences. *Am J Neuroradiol* 1995;16:281–288.

Weinberger E, Shaw DW, White KS, et al. Nontraumatic pediatric musculoskeletal MR imaging: comparison of conventional and fast-spin-echo short inversion time inversion-recovery technique. *Radiology* 1995;194:721–726.

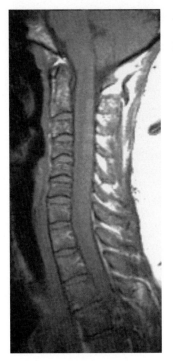

FIGURE 51.1

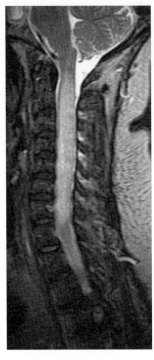

FIGURE 51.2

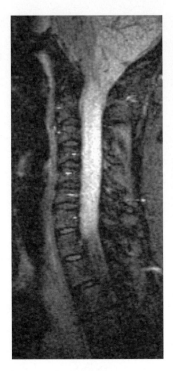

FIGURE 51.3

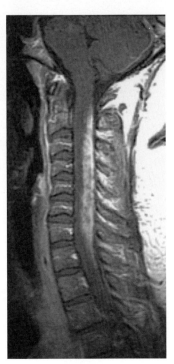

FIGURE 51.4

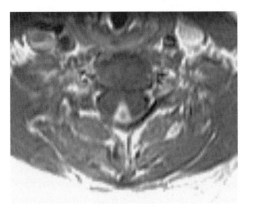

FIGURE 51.5

HISTORY

A 52-year-old African-American female with a burning sensation in her hands and feet.

FINDINGS

Sagittal T1-weighted image (Fig. 51.1) shows marked and diffuse cervical cord enlargement. The sagittal T2-weighted fast spin echo (Fig. 51.2) and the sagittal fast short inversion time inversion-recovery (STIR) (Fig. 51.3) image show dif-fuse high signal intensity throughout the substance of the en-larged cord spanning the C1 through the T7 level. Follow-ing contrast administration, the sagittal (Fig. 51.4) and axial (Fig. 51.5) T1-weighted images show marked enhancement within the dorsal aspect of the cord in the midline, involving the dorsal columns bilaterally. The enhancement extends to the cord surface and deep in the midline. The pattern appears to be both leptomeningeal and intramedullary.

DIAGNOSIS

Sarcoidosis.

DISCUSSION

Sarcoidosis is a multisystem, noncaseating, granulomatous disease. Clinical involvement of the central nervous system (CNS) is seen in approximately 5% of cases. It most commonly involves the basal meninges, cranial nerves, hypothalamus, and pituitary gland. The spinal cord and adjacent spinal meninges are rarely involved. Of the histologically proven cases, 35% are predominantly intramedullary, 35% extramedullary, and 23% both. Extradural involvement has been reported in less than 2%. On imaging studies, an intramedullary mass lesion in the cervical or upper thoracic cord was the most common finding.

Although both the cord and meninges are often involved together in a patchy distribution, the most common finding on imaging studies is cord widening, an obviously nonspecific finding. Contrast-enhanced MR greatly increases the sensitivity of MR for detecting both intramedullary and leptomeningeal sarcoid. If seen together, this may suggest sarcoid rather than an intrameduallary neoplasm and obviate the need for biopsy of the cord and excision. A postulated theory as to why sarcoid affects both the leptomeninges and cord is that the cord parenchyma is secondarily involved by spread through the superficial perivascular spaces from the leptomeninges.

BIBLIOGRAPHY

Atkinson R, Ghelman B, Tsairis P, et al. Sarcoidosis presenting as cervical radiculopathy: a case report and literature review. *Spine* 1982;7:412–416.

Graf M, Wakhloo A, Schmidtke K, et al. Sarcoidosis of the spinal cord and medulla oblongata: a pathological and neuroradiological case report. *Clin Neuropathol* 1994;13:19–25.

Lexa FJ, Grossman RI. MR of sarcoidosis in the head and spine: spectrum of manifestations and radiographic response to steroid therapy. *Am J Neuroradiol* 1994;15:973–982.

Miller DH, Kendall BE, Barter S, et al. Magnetic resonance imaging in central nervous system sarcoidosis. *Neurology* 1988;38:378–383.

Pascuzzi RM, Shapiro SA, Rau AN, et al. Sarcoid myelopathy. *J Neuroimaging* 1996;6:61–62.

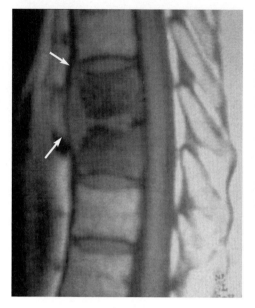

FIGURE 52.1

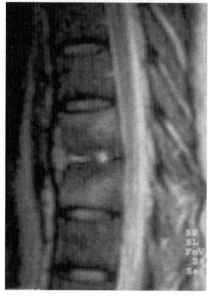

FIGURE 52.2

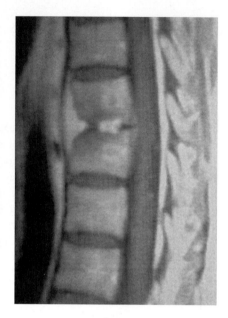

FIGURE 52.3

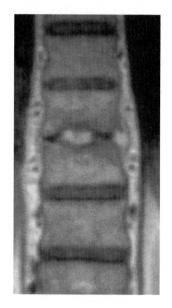

FIGURE 52.4

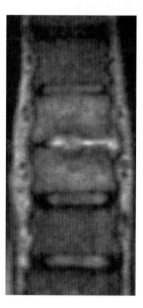

FIGURE 52.5

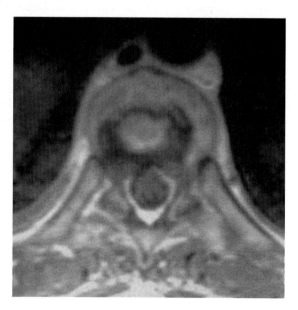

FIGURE 52.6

HISTORY

A 33-year-old with low back pain.

FINDINGS

Sagittal T1-weighted through the midthoracic spine (Fig. 52.1) and the sagittal fast spin echo T2 images (Fig. 52.2) show abnormal signal intensity involving two adjacent vertebral bodies in the intervening intervertebral disk.

There is irregularity of the end plates. The disk itself and the vertebral body show high signal intensity on the T2-weighted image. Soft-tissue mass extends anteriorly along the vertebral bodies with irregularity of the anterior margins of the vertebral bodies. The soft-tissue mass appears delineated by the anterior longitudinal ligament (*arrows*). Following contrast material, the sagittal T1-weighted image (Fig. 52.3) and the coronal T1-weighted image (Fig. 52.4) show enhancement within the substance of the vertebral disk, as well as enhancement of the soft-tissue mass along the anterior margin of the vertebral body and un-derneath the anterior longitudinal ligament. A small amount of posterior extension is seen into the anterior epidural space without evidence of cord compromise. Coronal T2-weighted image (Fig. 52.5) also shows high signal intensity within the intervertebral disk extending into the left side of the disk and paravertebral space, and also high signal within both vertebral bodies. Axial T1-weighted image following contrast (Fig. 52.6) shows the central abnormal enhancement and lack of significant mass effect upon the cord. Images courtesy of Joseph Illes, Johannesburg, South Africa.

DIAGNOSIS

Tuberculous spondylitis.

DISCUSSION

The most common form of skeletal tuberculosis (TB) is spinal TB. Its incidence is increasing primarily because of the emergence of AIDS; thus the awareness of its MR imaging features has become more important. The diagnosis is often difficult because the onset of TB spondylitis is insidious and its course is more indolent than pyogenic infection. Typically, TB spondylitis begins in the anterior inferior portion of the vertebral body. Infection classically spreads beneath the anterior longitudinal ligament to involve contiguous or noncontiguous vertebral bodies. The amount of bony destruction relative to degree of disk involvement is usually greater than that seen with pyogenic infection, which can lead to the characteristic gibbus deformity. In fact, the disk space may be uninvolved and the disk signal may be normal on T2-weighted images. Posterior element involvement is more common than in other infections. Isolated posterior element or vertebral body involvement may lead to confusion with tumor and consequent delays in instituting proper therapy. In these cases, tissue sampling is the only means of diagnosis as the clinical and MR findings are nonspecific. Large paraspinal masses out of proportion to the amount of bone destruction, which often calcify, are more common with TB spondylitis.

A variety of less common fungal and nontuberculous granulomatous infections can also occur in the spine that can appear similar to TB spondylitis. Uncommon entities such as pseudoarthrosis associated with ankylosing spondylitis and hemodialysis-associated spondyloarthropathy may also mimic disk space infection and should be considered in the appropriate clinical context.

BIBLIOGRAPHY

Ahmadi J, Baja JA, Destian S, et al. Spinal tuberculosis: atypical observations at MR imaging. *Radiology* 1993;189:489.

Del COJ, Gower DJ, McWhorter JM. Changing concepts in spinal epidural abscess: a report of 29 cases. *Neurosurgery* 1990;27:185–192.

Sharif HS, Aideyan OA, Clark DC, et al. Brucellar and tuberculous spondylitis: comparative imaging features. *Radiology* 1989;171:419–425.

Smith AJ, Weinstein MA, Mizushmia A, et al. MR imaging characteristics of tuberculous spondylitis vs. vertebral osteomyelitis. *Am J Neuroradiol* 1989;10:619.

Wurtz R, Quader Z, Simon D, et al. Cervical tuberculous vertebral osteomyelitis: case report and discussion of the literature. *Clin Infect Dis* 1993;16:806–808.

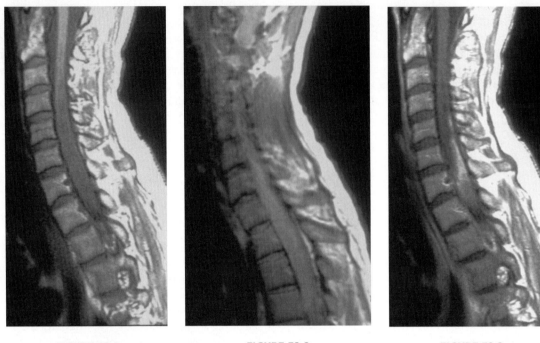

FIGURE 53.1   FIGURE 53.2   FIGURE 53.3

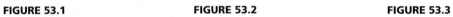

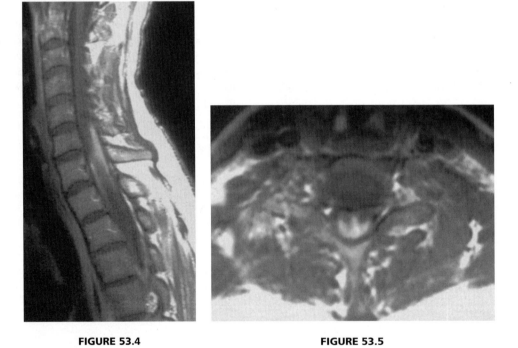

FIGURE 53.4   FIGURE 53.5

HISTORY

A 42-year-old with rapid onset of leg weakness progressing to flaccid paralysis.

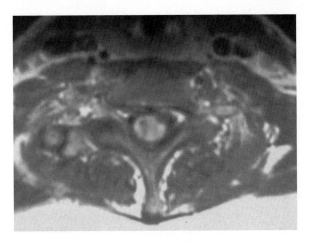

FIGURE 53.6

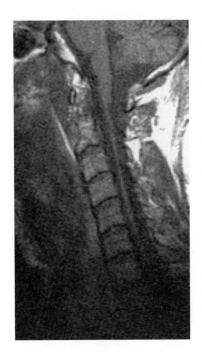

FIGURE 53.7

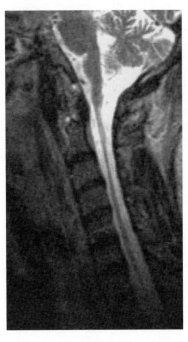

FIGURE 53.8

FINDINGS

Sagittal T1-weighted image without contrast (Fig. 53.1) shows diffuse and fusiform cord enlargement involving the cervical spine inferior to the C3–4 level. This shows high signal intensity on the sagittal spin density-weighted image (Fig. 53.2). This again is diffuse within the cervical thoracic cord. Two sagittal T1-weighted images (Figs. 53.3 and 53.4) show marked cord enhancement at the C6 through T1 levels. Enhancement appears along the cord surface but does extend deep into the substance of the cord itself. Two axial T1-weighted images following contrast (Fig. 53.5 and 53.6) also show the enhancement that involves the periphery of the cord but extends to involve both the central gray matter and adjacent white matter. Follow-up sagittal T1-weighted (Fig. 53.7) and sagittal T2-weighted fast spin echo (Fig. 53.8) images 2 years following the prior study show marked and diffuse cord atrophy.

DIAGNOSIS

Demyelinating disease.

DISCUSSION

Up to 20% of patients with demyelinating disease may exhibit only spinal cord abnormalities and not have MR-visible parenchymal brain lesions. Lesions may also occur within the cord in these patients that are asymptomatic. Acutely, demyelinating plaques can show cord enlargement and edema, and this may occasionally extend over several segments, as in this case. The enhancement pattern in this case is a clue to the diagnosis, since there is preferential enhancement along the periphery of the cord as well as more central patchy enhancement. Neoplasms such as a glioma or ependymoma are very unlikely to give such a linear pattern involving both the central aspect of the cord and its periphery. Because of the enhancement pattern this would fall more into an infectious/inflammatory category. Other differential considerations would include a viral or postviral demyelinating process, primary viral infection, and granulomatous processes such as sarcoidosis. Occasionally, the inciting demyelinating event will be more florid and could almost be considered as a tumefactive-type demyelination presenting within the cord. This case also shows the profound cord atrophy that can occur following such a devastating monophasic event.

BIBLIOGRAPHY

Filippi M, Yousry TA, Alkadhi H, et al. Spinal cord MRI in multiple sclerosis with multicoil arrays: a comparison between fast spin echo and fast FLAIR. *J Neurol Neurosurg Psychiatry* 1996;61:632–635.

Ford B, Tampieri D, Francis G. Long-term follow-up of acute partial transverse myelopathy. *Neurology* 1992;42:250–252.

Thorpe JW, Kidd D, Moseley IF, et al. Spinal MRI in patients with suspected multiple sclerosis and negative brain MRI. *Brain* 1996;119:709–714.

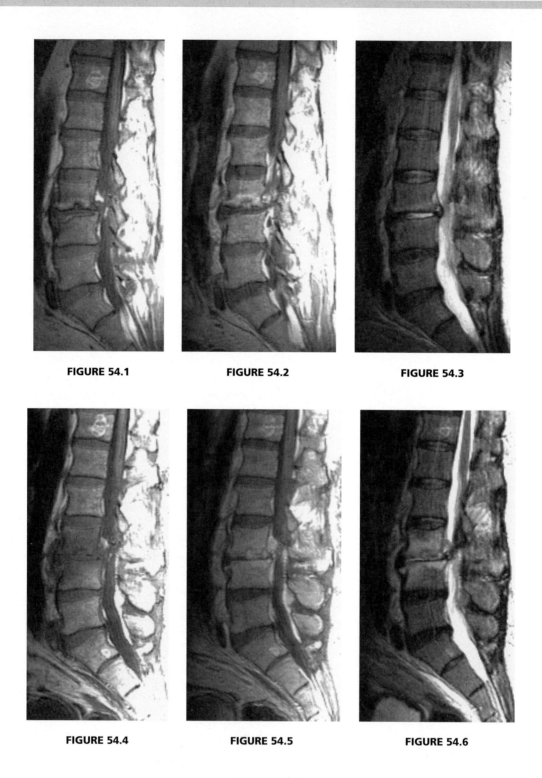

FIGURE 54.1   **FIGURE 54.2**   **FIGURE 54.3**

FIGURE 54.4   **FIGURE 54.5**   **FIGURE 54.6**

HISTORY

A 62-year-old with a history of recent enterococcal bacteremia, now with worsening back pain.

FINDINGS

Initial sagittal T1-weighted (Fig. 54.1), sagittal T1-weighted following contrast (Fig. 54.2), and sagittal fast spin echo T2-weighted image (Fig. 54.3) show loss of disk space height at the L3–4 level with a Schmorl's node involving inferior end plate of L3. There is enhancement of the inferior end plate of L3 that shows fatty marrow infiltration on the unenhanced image. The T2-weighted image shows linear high signal intensity within the intervertebral disk at L3–4 without significant high signal intensity within the adjacent vertebral bodies. There is a small disk extrusion at L3–4.

Follow-up exam 2 weeks later shows marked interval change, now showing irregularity and more flow signal intensity within the L3–4 bodies on the unenhanced T1-weighted images (Fig. 54.4). Following contrast administration, the sagittal T1-weighted image (Fig. 54.5) shows increased enhancement within the intervertebral disk proper, as well as increased soft tissue within the anterior epidural space consistent with phlegmon. Sagittal T2-weighted image (Fig. 54.6) also shows increased signal from the L3–4 bodies and high signal from the disk space itself.

DIAGNOSIS

Early disk space infection masked by degenerative end plate and disk disease.

DISCUSSION

Because of the often nonspecific symptoms, the clinical diagnosis of vertebral osteomyelitis is difficult, which in turn can contribute to a delay in diagnosis and subsequent increase in patient morbidity and mortality. MR imaging allows the early diagnosis of disk space infection and thus plays a critical role in both diagnosis and patient follow-up. There are several routes of spread of infection to the spine, the most common being hematogenous dissemination from an extraspinal primary source. Vertebral osteomyelitis may be classified into pyogenic (most commonly secondary to *Staphylococcus aureus*) and nonpyogenic (tuberculous or fungal) varieties.

Pyogenic vertebral osteomyelitis typically occurs in the sixth to seventh decade, although it can be seen in younger patients, especially intravenous drug abusers and those with HIV infection. The richly vascularized subchondral bone adjacent to the end plate is the most common site of initial infection, with subsequent spread into the intervertebral disk and adjacent vertebral body. Early findings of disk space infection are best depicted on T1-weighted sagittal images as abnormal low signal within the disk space and adjacent vertebral body marrow, with obscuration of the normal thin, linear, low-signal end plates. T2-weighted images reveal abnormal increased signal within the disk and adjacent marrow. As the infection progresses, the disk space becomes progressively narrowed and there is increasing destruction of the vertebral bodies. Varying patterns of enhancement can be seen within the infected vertebral bodies and disk space. However, straightforward cases of vertebral osteomyelitis do not require Gd-DTPA for diagnosis. Prevertebral and paraspinal inflammation is common, with occasional formation of a paraspinal abscess. Contrast is useful in distinguishing paraspinal abscesses from solid-tissue inflammation (phlegmon).

Epidural infection generally appears isointense to hypointense to neural elements on unenhanced T1-weighted images and variably hyperintense on T2-weighted images. Epidural infection is commonly associated with adjacent disk space infection, although occasionally primary epidural infection can be seen from hematogenous spread without adjacent vertebral body or disk infection. In this setting, contrast is valuable in characterizing epidural infection, helping to define its presence and extent, and in assisting in discrimination between the infection and the adjacent spinal canal contents. The pattern of contrast enhancement may also influence surgical management, as small, solid areas of enhancement without neurologic sequelae can be managed medically, whereas peripherally enhancing epidural collections generally require surgical evacuation.

BIBLIOGRAPHY

Dagirmanjian A, Schils J, McHenry M, et al. MR imaging of vertebral osteomyelitis revisited. *Am J Roentgenol* 1996;167:1539–1543.

Modic MT, Feiglin DH, Piraino DW, et al. Vertebral osteomyelitis: assessment using MR. *Radiology* 1985;157:157–166.

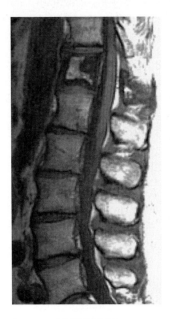

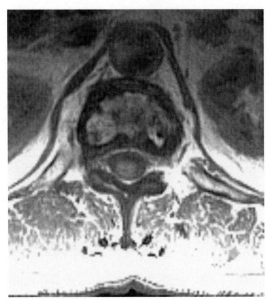

FIGURE 55.1   **FIGURE 55.2**

HISTORY

A 72-year-old with a history of prostate carcinoma, now with elevated PSA, and question of metastatic disease.

FINDINGS

Sagittal (Fig. 55.1) and axial (Fig. 55.2) T1-weighted images through the lumbar spine show a "picture frame" type of low signal intensity outlining the T12 vertebral body. There is also straightening of the cortical margins on the sagittal view. There is abnormal low signal intensity diffusely within the posterior elements at T12. The adjacent vertebral bodies and intervertebral disks are unremarkable. There is no evidence of associated soft-tissue mass. The T12 body shows central high signal intensity consistent with fatty marrow.

DIAGNOSIS

Paget's disease.

DISCUSSION

Osteitis deformans was first described by Sir James Paget in 1877 and continues to bear his name; however, the etiology of this common abnormality (3% of the population over 40 years) remains obscure. Viral, autoimmune, and genetic factors have all been implicated in the genesis of Paget's disease. It may be a localized process involving one or more bones and is often discovered incidentally; less commonly, it is more diffuse and may produce extensive osseous deformity. The axial skeleton is commonly affected, with frequent involvement of the pelvis (40%), spine (75%), and skull (65%). Local pain and tenderness are frequently present, and neurologic deficits (including motor weakness and incontinence) from spinal cord impingement may follow vertebral body compression fractures or bony expansion resulting from remodeling.

The disease is characterized by abnormal remodeling of bone, which produces a characteristic pathologic and radiographic appearance with irregular bony fragments that are visualized as coarsened and enlarged osseous trabeculae. Initially, resorption of bony trabeculae predominates because of the intense osteoclastic activity. This is recognized on radiographs as the osteolytic form of the disease, which is particularly common in the skull, where it is termed *osteoporosis circumscripta*. Subsequently, abnormal bone remodeling can occur, which results in enlargement of bone and cortical thickening due to bone apposition on the periosteal and endosteal envelopes. Increased external bone diameter with a thin cortex is caused by periosteal apposition with concomitant resorption along the endosteal envelope, leading to enlargement of the marrow cavity. Radiographic evidence of increased density or sclerosis of bone may be seen in both active and inactive stages of the disease.

The MR appearance of Paget's disease reflects not only the changes of abnormal bone remodeling but also the attendant changes in the vertebral body marrow space. In the active phases of the disease the hematopoietic bone marrow is replaced by fibrous connective tissue with large, numerous vascular channels. In the inactive (osteosclerotic) phases the marrow may revert to normal. Cystlike lesions representing fat-filled marrow cavities can be present. Blood-filled sinusoids and cystic areas can appear radiographically as lucencies and have also been described in Paget's disease. The MR appearance of Paget's disease includes cortical thickening, depicted as hypointense areas or areas of signal void on all pulse sequences. Focal regions of signal within the normal void of cortical bone may follow the introduction of cellular or other marrow elements during remodeling; within the medullary canal, signal can be highly variable. Areas of decreased signal intensity on short TR/TE images can also be seen, with increased intensity on long TR/TE that might be due to fibrovascular change in the marrow in active Paget's disease. The presence of hypointensity on short TR/TE images and hyperintensity on long TR/TE images, however, is nonspecific and, if associated with new-onset pain, should prompt consideration of pathologic fracture or sarcomatous degeneration.

BIBLIOGRAPHY

Bahk YW, Park YH, Chung SK, et al. Bone pathologic correlation of multimodality imaging in Paget's disease. *J Nucl Med* 1995;36:1421–1426.

Boutin RD, Spitz DJ, Newman JS, et al. Complications in Paget disease at MR imaging. *Radiology* 1998;209:641–651.

Mirra JM, Brien EW, Tehranzadeh J. Paget's disease of bone: review with emphasis on radiologic features, Part I. *Skeletal Radiol* 1995;24:163–171.

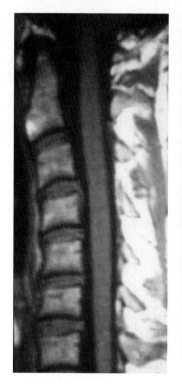

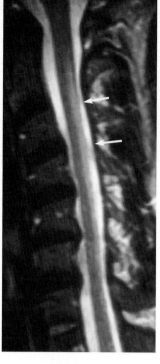

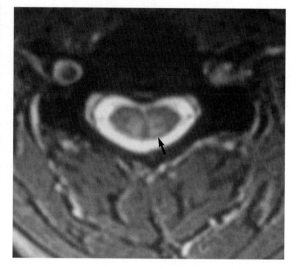

FIGURE 56.1   FIGURE 56.2   FIGURE 56.3

HISTORY

A 41-year-old with paresthesias and ataxia.

FINDINGS

Sagittal T1-weighted image (Fig. 56.1) is unremarkable. Sagittal T2-weighted image (Fig. 56.2) and the axial gradient echo image (Fig. 56.3) show abnormal well-defined increased signal intensity involving the dorsal aspect of the cervical cord just adjacent to the midline (*arrows*). This occurs over multiple segments and appears to involve the dorsal columns. There is no evidence of cord enlargement.

DIAGNOSIS

Subacute combined degeneration.

DISCUSSION

Subacute combined degeneration (SCD) is secondary to a deficiency of vitamin B12, which involves the brain and the optic and peripheral nerves. Vitamin B12 serves as a coenzyme in the reaction leading to the formation of myelin basic protein. Neuropathologic findings initially include swelling of the myelin sheaths, with little axon change in the posterior columns of the upper cervical segments. Later, the myelin sheath and axonal degeneration and loss are seen leading to Wallerian-type degeneration of the long tracts. Typical clinical presentations include paresthesias, stiffness, numbness or tingling of the limbs, and slight sensory ataxia and loss of posterior column function. Many conditions may produce vitamin B12 deficiency, such as inadequate intake and malabsorption. Pernicious anemia (megaloblastic anemia) following gastrectomy, intestinal infection, and ileal abnormalities may also produce this abnormality. Nitrous oxide administration can precipitate the occurrence of SCD in patients with borderline vitamin B12 deficiency by enhancing the oxidation of B12, rendering it ineffective. MR is the method of choice for showing the demyelination of the spinal cord, seen as increased signal in the T2-weighted images and a typical distribution of the dorsal and lateral columns. Axial imaging is very useful in precisely defining the location of the high signal abnormality on MR. Signal abnormalities may persist in the cord for up to a year following treatment and presumably reflects residual demyelination and/or gliosis.

BIBLIOGRAPHY

Berger JR, Quencer R. Reversible myelopathy with pernicious anemia: clinical/MR correlation. *Neurology* 1991;41:947–948.

Hemmer B, Glocker FX, Schumacher M, et al. Subacute combined degeneration: clinical, electrophysiological, and magnetic resonance imaging findings. *J Neurol Neurosurg Psychiatry* 1998;65:822–827.

Katsaros VK, Glocker FX, Hemmer B, et al. MRI of spinal cord and brain lesions in subacute combined degeneration. *Neuroradiology* 1998;40:716–719.

Locatelli ER, Laureno R, Ballard P, et al. MRI in vitamin B12 deficiency myelopathy. *Can J Neurol Sci* 1999;26:60–63.

Sharma S, Khilnani GC, Berry M. Case of the season: megaloblastic anemia with subacute combined degeneration (SCD) of the spinal cord. *Semin Roentgenol* 1999;34:2–4.

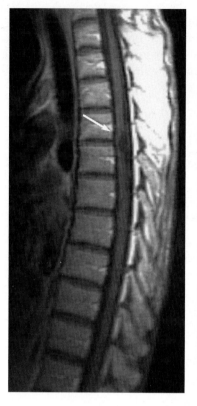 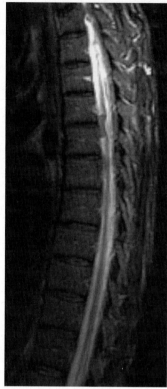 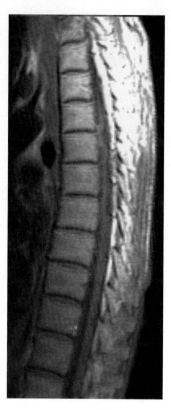

FIGURE 57.1   **FIGURE 57.2**   **FIGURE 57.3**

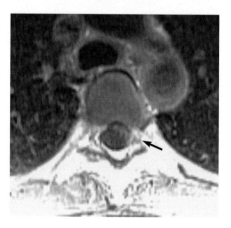

FIGURE 57.4

HISTORY

A 47-year-old with gradual onset of myelopathy.

FINDINGS

Sagittal T1-weighted image in the midline (Fig. 57.1) shows an apparent "defect" in the dorsal aspect of the tho-racic cord which is hugging the anterior margins of the dura and posterior margin of the vertebral bodies (*arrow*). Left parasagittal fast spin echo T2 image (Fig. 57.2) and the corresponding sagittal T1-weighted image (Fig. 57.3) show an abrupt transition from normal cord into the cord that is abutting the posterior margins of the vertebral bodies. No abnormal signal is seen within this segment. Axial T1-weighted image through that level (Fig. 57.4) shows the small cord, which is displaced anteriorly and to the left within the left thecal sac (*arrow*). There is a slight irregularity along the right ventral margin of the thecal sac, which is assuming a more "dumbbell" configuration.

DIAGNOSIS

Idiopathic spinal cord herniation.

DISCUSSION

Symptomatic anterior dural herniation of the spinal cord is a rare entity that is surgically treatable. The lesion can produce a Brown-Sequard syndrome or a spastic paraparesis. Although uncommon, it does have a very distinctive imaging appearance that allows unequivocal diagnosis. The most important points of this entity include the typical presentation as Brown-Sequard syndrome, that the clinical deficit tends to be progressive and less treated, and that surgical reduction of the herniated cord can lead to improvement in the motor deficit. The typical patient is an adult, with the typical affected location of the upper and midthoracic level (T2–T7). It tends to occur on the left anterolateral dura. Patients often present with a long history of subtle hemisensory abnormality before the motor symptoms begin. MR is very useful and shows a typical pattern of an interruption of the usually smooth ventral margin of the cord being thrust anteriorly over a very short segment. Primary differential is whether this is being displaced from a posterior mass such as arachnoid cyst or whether the cord is being tethered ventrally. Then axial sections may be allowed this distinction or CT myelography through this area. The etiology of this abnormality is unclear. Many theories have been advanced, including herniation into a preexisting ventral meningocele; unrecognized traumatic event causing a ventral dural disruption; intrathecal rupture of thoracic disk, creating a dural defect; or preexisting congenital ventral dural defect.

BIBLIOGRAPHY

Borges LF, Zervas NT, Lehrich JR. Idiopathic spinal cord herniation: a treatable cause of the Brown-Sequard syndrome—case report. *Neurosurgery* 1995;36:1028–1032.

Dix JE, Griffitt W, Yates C, et al. Spontaneous thoracic spinal cord herniation through an anterior dural defect. *Am J Neuroradiol* 1998;19:1345–1348.

Hausmann ON, Moseley IF. Idiopathic dural herniation of the thoracic spinal cord. *Neuroradiology* 1996;38:503–510.

Sioutos P, Arbit E, Tsairis P, et al. Spontaneous thoracic spinal cord herniation: a case report. *Spine* 1996;21:1710–1713.

Watters MR, Stears JC, Osborn AG, et al. Transdural spinal cord herniation: imaging and clinical spectra. *Am J Neuroradiol* 1998;19:1337–1344.

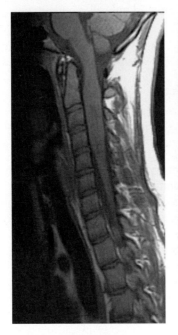 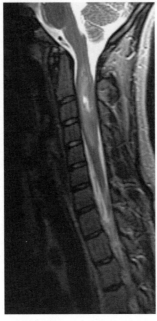 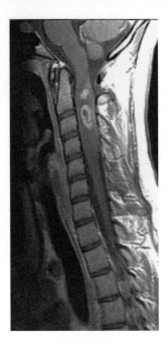

FIGURE 58.1 **FIGURE 58.2** **FIGURE 58.3**

HISTORY

A 39-year-old with leg and arm weakness.

FINDINGS

Sagittal T1-weighted image (Fig. 58.1) shows fusiform enlargement of the cervical cord from the C2 through the C4–5 level. The sagittal fast spin echo T2-weighted image (Fig. 58.2) shows high signal intensity with fairly well-defined margins from the cervical cord. A more focal area of high signal is seen centrally within the cord at the C3 level. Following contrast administration, the sagittal T1-weighted image (Fig. 58.3) shows areas of irregular and ring enhancement at the C2–3 levels.

DIAGNOSIS

Glioma.

DISCUSSION

Gliomas are the predominant intramedullary tumor and may be subclassified into ependymomas, astrocytomas, glioblastomas, and oligodendrogliomas. Ependymomas are the most common, accounting for approximately 63% of spinal gliomas. They are vascular tumors and are more likely to bleed when compared with other intramedullary tumors. The archetypal tumor patient was middle-aged and male

(1.3:1 predilection), with tumors occurring equally in the thoracic area and cervical cord, involving fewer than four vertebral body segments. The patient had clinical symptoms of pain, radiculopathy, sensory or motor deficits, and incontinence.

T1-weighted images typically demonstrate fusiform widening of the cord over one or several segments by a soft-tissue mass that is isointense or slightly hypointense to normal cord. T2-weighted images demonstrate focal areas of increased signal within the enlarged cord segments that represent the tumor and surrounding edema. There is a frequent association of both intratumoral cysts and an adjacent syrinx with astrocytomas (38%) and ependymomas (45%). It is difficult to differentiate cystic tumor from a benign or adjacent syrinx on standard spin echo sequences, because the signal may vary, depending on the fluid characteristics. Contrast may help in this regard, because all gliomas can be expected to enhance. A reliable differentiation between ependymoma and astrocytoma cannot be made on the basis of MR characteristics in the cervical and thoracic cord. The differential diagnosis of intramedullary gliomas should include metastases, hemangioblastomas, and embryonal tumors, as well as nonneoplastic, cystic-appearing lesions that enlarge the cord, such as syringohydromyelia, transverse myelitis, tumefactive multiple sclerosis abscess, ependymal cyst, and hematomas. Histologic type is a significant predictor of survival in patients with astrocytoma of the spinal cord, with the 10-year overall survival rate 81% for patients with pilocytic astrocytoma, compared with 15% for those with diffuse fibrillary astrocytoma. The survival rate is highest in patients who undergo biopsy followed by postoperative radiation therapy. The extent of surgical resection (biopsy versus subtotal resection versus gross total resection) is a much less significant predictor of survival among patients with pilocytic or nonpilocytic astrocytomas of the spinal cord.

BIBLIOGRAPHY

Bouffet E, Pierre-Kahn A, Marchal JC, et al. Prognostic factors in pediatric spinal cord astrocytoma. *Cancer* 1998;83:2391–2399.

Bourgouin PM, Lesage J, Fontaine S, et al. A pattern approach to the differential diagnosis of intramedullary spinal cord lesions on MR imaging. *Am J Roentgenol* 1998;170:1645–1649.

Steinbok P. Spinal cord astrocytomas: long-term results comparing treatments in children. *Childs Nerv Syst* 1998;14:1.

Sze G. MR imaging of the spinal cord: current status and future advances. *Am J Roentgenol* 1992;159:149–159.

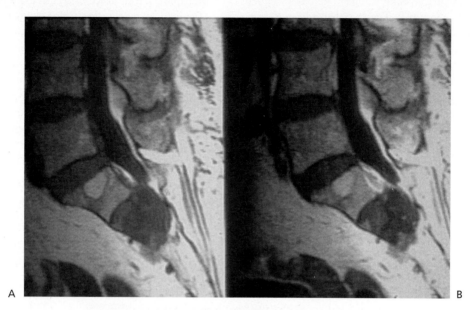

FIGURE 59.1

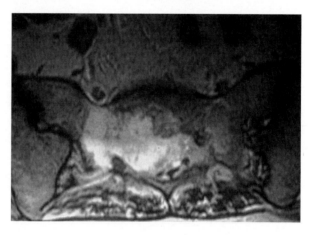

FIGURE 59.2

HISTORY

A 50-year-old with low back pain.

FINDINGS

Sagittal T1-weighted image without contrast (Fig. 59.1A) shows a well-defined mass of low signal intensity involving the S2 vertebral body, with extension into the caudal epidural space. Following contrast administration, the sagittal T1-weighted image (Fig. 59.1B) shows very mild enhancement. Axial T2-weighted image (Fig. 59.2) shows high signal intensity coming from the mass.

DIAGNOSIS

Chordoma.

DISCUSSION

Chordoma is a tumor arising from notachordal rests and represents approximately 3% to 5% of primary bone tumors. It is most frequently found in the sacrococcygeal region (50%). Other sites include the clivus (35%) and the vertebral column (15%). The cervical and lumbar regions are more frequently involved than the thoracic area. The tumor is locally aggressive and rarely metastasizes. Chordoma may involve two adjacent vertebral bodies and the intervening disk, an unusual feature of spinal tumors. MR findings include a large paravertebral or presacral soft-tissue mass, which may be much larger than expected from the amount of bone involvement. T1 images demonstrate isointensity (75%) or hypointensity (25%) with bone destruction. Nonspecific increased signal is seen on T2-weighted images. These are low-signal septations in a majority of cases. Magnetic resonance imaging is superior to CT in determining the extent and relationship of the tumor to neural structures, but CT better shows bone destruction and calcification.

BIBLIOGRAPHY

Boriani S, Chevalley F, Weinstein JN, et al. Chordoma of the spine above the sacrum: treatment and outcome in 21 cases. *Spine* 1996;21:1569–1577.

Firooznia H, Pinto RS, Lin JP, et al. Chordoma: radiologic evaluation of 20 cases. *Am J Roentgenol* 1976;127:797–805.

Murphey MD, Andrews CL, Flemming DJ, et al. From the archives of the AFIP. Primary tumors of the spine: radiologic pathologic correlation. *Radiographics* 1996;16:1131–1158.

Sze G, Uichanco LS, Brant-Zawadzki MN, et al. Chordomas: MR imaging. *Radiology* 1988;166:187–191.

Weber AL, Liebsch NJ, Sanchez R, et al. Chordomas of the skull base: radiologic and clinical evaluation. *Neuroimaging Clin North Am* 1994;4:515–527.

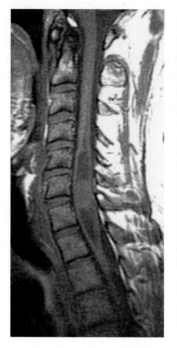

FIGURE 60.1

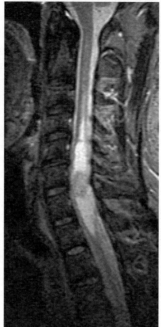

FIGURE 60.2

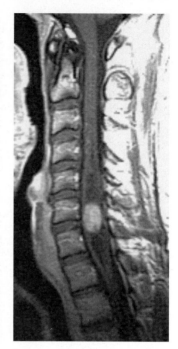

FIGURE 60.3

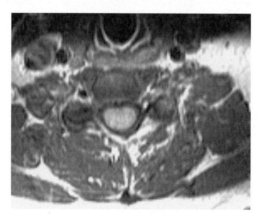

FIGURE 60.4

HISTORY

A 36-year-old with gradual onset of arm and leg numbness.

FINDINGS

Sagittal T1-weighted image without contrast (Fig. 60.1) shows fusiform enlargement of the cervical cord from levels C4–5 through T1. There is central low signal intensity, with a rounded area of soft-tissue signal within the lesion. The sagittal T2-weighted image (Fig. 60.2) shows that the areas of low signal on the T1 image now show high signal consistent with fluid. The central soft-tissue signal now is nearly isointense to cord. Following contrast administration, the sagittal (Fig. 60.3) and axial (Fig. 60.4) T1-weighted images show marked enhancement of the focal central nidus at the C6–7 level. No additional cord enhancement is seen. No flow void is identified to suggest feeding vessels.

DIAGNOSIS

Ependymoma.

DISCUSSION

Gliomas are the most common intramedullary spinal cord tumor, of which ependymomas account for approximately 63%. They are relatively slow growing and may expand the spinal canal, especially when located in the filum or conus. They are associated with cystic degeneration in 45% of cases. A large percentage can arise in the lumbar and sacral regions (37% to 51%) and may arise from the filum, with a small percentage (3%) involving the extradural portion of the filum. The second most common glioma of the cord is an astrocytoma, with benign grades representing the majority. They are associated with cyst formation in 38%. Focal astrocytomas involve the thoracic cord most commonly, with cervical involvement second; they tend to be more extensive than ependymomas, involving several levels and occasionally the entire cord.

Intramedullary ependymomas are characterized by focal enlargement of the cord and decreased signal on T1-weighted images, and increased signal on T2-weighted images. They are well-circumscribed, enhancing masses. Contrast-enhanced MR is useful to identify and localize primary tumor, as well as recurrence and seeding along the neural axis (factors that could be missed on plain MR alone). The use of enhanced MR permits differentiation of ependymoma from peritumoral reactive cysts, postoperative changes, or changes resulting from prior radiation therapy. However, enhancement of these tumors is quite variable, and no enhancement may occur.

BIBLIOGRAPHY

Bourgouin PM, Lesage J, Fontaine S, et al. A pattern approach to the differential diagnosis of intramedullary spinal cord lesions on MR imaging. *Am J Roentgenol* 1998;170:1645–1649.

Fine MJ, Kricheff II, Freed D, et al. Spinal cord ependymomas: MR imaging features. *Radiology* 1995;197:655–658.

Kahan H, Sklar EM, Post MJ, et al. MR characteristics of histopathologic subtypes of spinal ependymoma. *Am J Neuroradiol* 1996;17:143–150.

Lefton DR, Pinto RS, Martin SW. MRI features of intracranial and spinal ependymomas. *Pediatr Neurosurg* 1998;28:97–105.

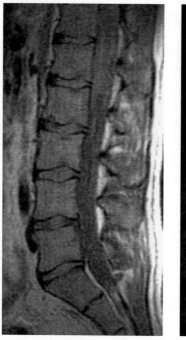

FIGURE 61.1

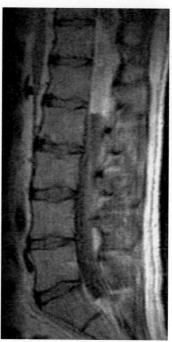

FIGURE 61.2

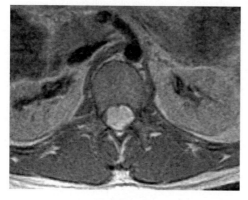

FIGURE 61.3

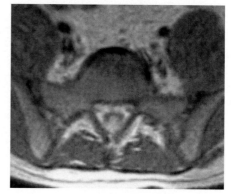

FIGURE 61.4

HISTORY

A 49-year-old with back pain and leg weakness.

FINDINGS

Sagittal T1-weighted images before contrast (Fig. 61.1) and after contrast (Fig. 61.2) show a very-ill-defined mass at the thoracolumbar junction. This does appear intradural following contrast administration and shows homogeneous and rather intense enhancement. Axial images at the thoracolumbar junction and at the S1 level following contrast administration (Figs. 61.3 and 61.4, respectively) show the primary intradural enhancing lesion as well as the second focus of abnormal enhancement within the caudal thecal sac. This enhancement can also be identified on the sagittal T1-weighted image following contrast.

DIAGNOSIS

Ependymoma.

DISCUSSION

Spinal ependymomas are benign, slow-growing tumors that arise from the ependymal lining of the central canal. Ependymomas account for at least 60% of spinal cord gliomas. Sixty percent of ependymomas occur in the conus medullaris/cauda equina region. Intradural extramedullary ependymomas of the spinal cord region are rare. Secondary intradural extramedullary lesions may result from cerebrospinal fluid spread. Intramedullary ependymomas are characterized by focal enlargement of the cord and low T1, and high T2 signal relative to normal cord. They are well-circumscribed masses showing variable enhancement. Contrast-enhanced MR is useful to identify and localize primary tumor, as well as recurrence and seeding along the neural axis. The use of enhanced MR permits differentiation of ependymoma from peritumoral reactive cysts, postoperative changes, or changes resulting from prior radiation therapy.

BIBLIOGRAPHY

Bourgouin PM, Lesage J, Fontaine S, et al. A pattern approach to the differential diagnosis of intramedullary spinal cord lesions on MR imaging. *Am J Roentgenol* 1998;170:1645–1649.

Fine MJ, Kricheff II, Freed D, et al. Spinal cord ependymomas: MR imaging features. *Radiology* 1995;197:655–658.

Kahan H, Sklar EM, Post MJ, et al. MR characteristics of histopathologic subtypes of spinal ependymoma. *Am J Neuroradiol* 1996;17:143–150.

Lefton DR, Pinto RS, Martin SW. MRI features of intracranial and spinal ependymomas. *Pediatr Neurosurg* 1998;28:97–105.

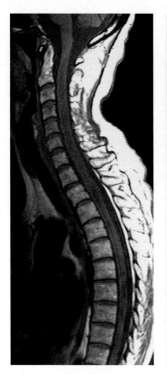 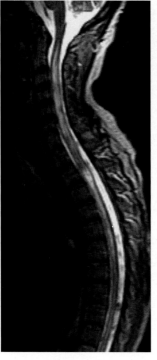 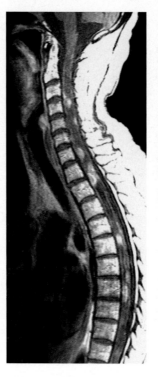 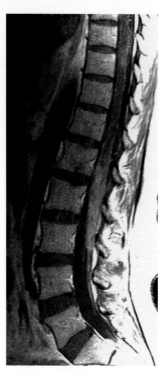

FIGURE 62.1   **FIGURE 62.2**   **FIGURE 62.3**   **FIGURE 62.4**

HISTORY

A 68-year-old with lung carcinoma, now with myelopathy.

FINDINGS

Sagittal T1-weighted image before contrast (Fig. 62.1) shows diffuse but mild enlargement of the cervical and thoracic cord, which also shows mild decreased signal intensity throughout. Sagittal T2-weighted image (Fig. 62.2) shows diffuse abnormal increased signal intensity involving the cervical and thoracic cord in a rather patchy fashion.

Following contrast administration, the sagittal T1-weighted images in the cervical (Fig. 62.3) and thoracolumbar region (Fig. 62.4) show a mixture of intramedullary enhancement, diffuse leptomeningeal enhancement along the cord periphery, and coating of the cauda equina.

DIAGNOSIS

Cord and leptomeningeal metastases.

DISCUSSION

The sites of leptomeningeal metastatic disease include two main areas, either from a CNS primary or from a systemic primary. Most common intracranial primaries causing spinal intradural metastasis are glioblastomas, primitive neuroectodermal tumors, and ependymomas. As in most other areas, primary systemic tumor types to metastasize are lung and breast carcinoma. Melanoma, lymphoma, and leukemias may also seed the CSF. Unenhanced imaging may be quite nonspecific, although with more involved cases where there is leptomeningeal and cord involvement, this may manifest as high signal intensity on the spin density or T2-weighted images within the cord. Following contrast, there is a typical "leptomeningeal" pattern of nodular and linear enhancement along the cord surface. As the tumor extends into the cord parenchyma, there can be more focal nodular enhancement.

This case shows a pattern of focal nodular intramedullary enhancement and more linear enhancement along the surface of the cord that would be consistent with leptomeningeal disease. This case would be useful to compare with Case 36, where diffuse enhancement relates to demyelinating disease. The distinctions are subtle, but the leptomeningeal tumor enhancement shows better-defined nodular areas of enhancement, where the demyelinating disease tends to be slightly patchy and more ill defined. However, when there is diffuse enhancement, distinction between granulomatous, demyelinating, postinfectious primary viral infection and tumor can be quite difficult.

BIBLIOGRAPHY

Dunne JW, Harper CG, Pamphlett R. Intramedullary spinal cord metastases: a clinical and pathological study of nine cases. *Q J Med* 1986;61:1003–1020.

Sze G, Krol G, Zimmerman RD, et al. Intramedullary disease of the spine: diagnosis using gadolinium-DTPA-enhanced MR imaging. *Am J Roentgenol* 1988;151:1193–1204.

Tognetti F, Lanzino G, Calbucci F. Metastases of the spinal cord from remote neoplasms: study of five cases. *Surg Neurol* 1988;30:220–227.

Winkelman MD, Adelstein DJ, Karlins NL. Intramedullary spinal cord metastasis: diagnostic and therapeutic considerations. *Arch Neurol* 1987;44:526–531.

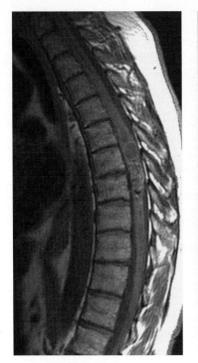

FIGURE 63.1

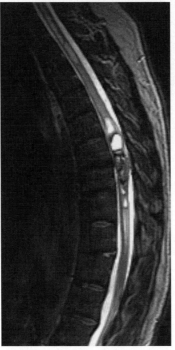

FIGURE 63.2

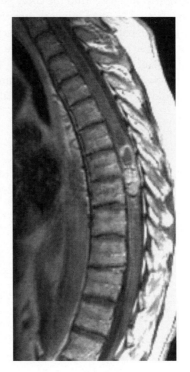

FIGURE 63.3

HISTORY

A 46-year-old with thoracic-level gradual-onset myelopathy.

FINDINGS

Sagittal T1-weighted image prior to contrast (Fig. 63.1) shows fusiform enlargement of the midthoracic cord. There is very heterogeneous signal intensity within the cord showing areas of focally low signal and other areas more superiorly with well-defined margins suggesting cysts. Slightly increased signal intensity is seen within the inferior aspect of the lesion. On the T2-weighted image (Fig. 63.2) there is also very heterogeneous signal intensity with areas of marked low signal intensity that could either reflect hemorrhage, calcification or other paramagnetic effects, and more superior cysts. Following contrast administration, the sagittal T1-weighted image (Fig. 63.3) shows focal areas of enhancement, with an area of ring enhancement along the superior margin. A syrinx is present within the upper thoracic and lower cervical cord that does not show abnormal enhancement following contrast administration.

DIAGNOSIS

Melanocytoma.

DISCUSSION

Melanocytomas are rare pigmented tumors of the central nervous system. The term *meningeal melanocytoma* was first reported in 1972 by Limas and Tio as a primary melanocytic from the leptomeninges with benign clinical and pathologic features. Melanocytes are widely distributed throughout the leptomeninges and occur in the highest concentration just ventrolateral to the medulla. Although the highest concentration of melanocytes occurs in the spinal leptomeninges in the upper cervical level, spinal meningeal melanocytomas are not confined to the cervical level and have been described as far as a thoracolumbar junction. These lesions can present involving the filum terminale or the cord surface, or they can present as an intradural extramedullary lesion similar to a meningioma. From an imaging standpoint, most of these lesions have been described as an intradural extramedullary mass. They can be locally invasive, however. MR imaging may be similar to the appearance of a meningioma, being isointense on T1- and diminished on T2-weighted images, and enhancing homogeneously. Histologic diagnosis may be difficult, and differential would include a malignant melanoma, a pigmented meningioma, and pigmented schwannoma. These lesions are dark brown or coal black at gross pathology, and microscopically are hypercellular tumors with cytoplasmic melanin pigment and prominent nucleoli. Mitotic figures should be rare or absent. In all, prognosis for patients with meningeal melanocytoma is good, with patients surviving at least several years after diagnosis. Local recurrence is common, however.

BIBLIOGRAPHY

Alameda F, Lloreta J, Galito E, et al. Meningeal melanocytoma: a case report and literature review. *Ultrastruct Pathol* 1998;22:349–356.

Clarke DB, Leblanc R, Bertrand G, et al. Meningeal melanocytoma: report of a case and a historical comparison. *J Neurosurg* 1998;88:116–121.

Czarnecki EJ, Silbergleit R, Gutierrez JA. MR of spinal meningeal melanocytoma. *Am J Neuroradiol* 1997;18:180–182.

Limas C, Tio Fo. Meningeal melanocytoma ("melanotic meningioma"). Its melanocytic origin as revealed by electron microscopy. *Cancer* 1972;30(5):1286–1294.

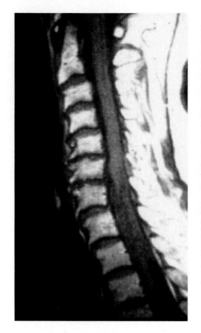

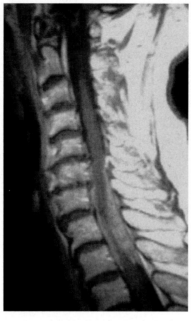

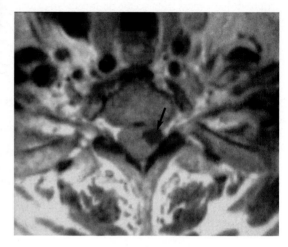

| FIGURE 64.1 | FIGURE 64.2 | FIGURE 64.3 |

HISTORY

A 61-year-old with gradual onset of leg weakness.

FINDINGS

Sagittal T1-weighted image (Fig. 64.1) has been windowed to more clearly show the low signal intensity margin of the cervical cord starting at the C6–7 level and extending inferiorly into the upper thoracic canal. The cord is indistinct at this level, and it is difficult to determine whether the abnormality is intra- or extradural. Sagittal T1-weighted images following contrast (Fig. 64.2) show enhancement along the margins of the cord at this level, both ventral and dorsal. The inferior margin shows a relatively obtuse angle with the dura but does suggest an intradural extramedullary process. This is confirmed on the axial T1-weighted image following contrast (Fig. 64.3) showing the cord being compressed and displaced to the left (*arrow*) and being surrounded by a diffuse enhancing tumor. The tumor is bounded peripherally by the dura and is clearly intradural.

DIAGNOSIS

Meningioma.

DISCUSSION

Intradural extramedullary neoplasms comprise the largest single group of primary spine neoplasms, accounting for approximately 55% of all primary spine tumors. The great majority of these tumors are benign, with nerve sheath tumors and meningiomas representing the most common lesions. The clinical presentation of intradural extramedullary tumors is often nonspecific. Local pain or radicular symptoms are the most common complaints, which can mimic disk herniation or other nonneoplastic processes. Nerve sheath tumors are the most common intraspinal tumors and are divided histologically into two types: schwannomas (also known as *neuromas, neurinomas,* and *neurilemomas*) and neurofibromas. This often confusing distinction is clinically important. Solitary schwannomas comprise the majority of intraspinal nerve sheath tumors, whereas neurofibromas are almost always associated with neurofibromatosis type I. Patients with neurofibromatosis type II, however, more commonly have multiple schwannomas rather than neurofibromas. Isolated nerve sheath tumors can arise anywhere in the spine. A small percentage are combined intradural-extradural (dumbbell shaped) or solely extradural. They typically occur in adults in their third through fifth decades, without any sex predilection.

Nerve sheath tumors are easily recognized on MR imaging as typically isolated, well-circumscribed, solid masses of soft-tissue signal intensity on T1-weighted images surrounded by low-signal CSF. On T2-weighted images they are of variable signal intensity. Schwannomas are more vascular and undergo cystic degeneration, necrosis, and hemorrhage more commonly than neurofibromas. Enhancement is variable, reflecting the underlying histologic changes. Malignant nerve sheath tumors are uncommon and are most commonly seen in patients with neurofibromatosis. They may arise *de novo* or from a preexisting nerve sheath tumor. Although malignant nerve sheath tumors more commonly are larger, are more inhomogeneous, and have more irregular margins, significant overlap with benign lesions precludes reliable distinction with current MR techniques. Meningiomas most commonly occur in the thoracic spine. As is the case intracranially, there is a female sex predilection, and these lesions occur in a slightly older age group than nerve sheath tumors. The great majority are entirely intradural and typically are isointense to the neural elements on T1- and T2-weighted images. Meningiomas enhance intensely after contrast administration, which may allow demonstration of the broad dural base. Calcification may render these lesions hypointense on all sequences.

BIBLIOGRAPHY

Edelhoff JC, Bates DJ, Ross JS, et al. Spinal MR findings in neurofibromatosis type 1 and 2. *Am J Neuroradiol* 1992;13:1071.

McCormick PC, Post KD, Stein BM. Intradural extramedullary tumors in adults. *Neurosurg Clin North Am* 1990;1:591.

Roux FX, Nataf F, Pinaudeau M, et al. Intraspinal meningiomas: review of 54 cases with discussion of poor prognosis factors and modern therapeutic management. *Surg Neurol* 1996;46:458–463.

Sevick RJ. Cervical spine tumors. *Neuroimaging Clin North Am* 1995;5:385–400.

Sze G, Abramson A, Krol G, et al. Gadolinium-DTPA in the evaluation of intradural extramedullary spinal disease. *Am J Roentgenol* 1988;150:911–921.

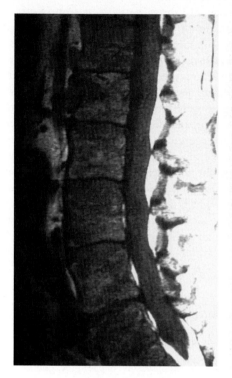

FIGURE 65.1

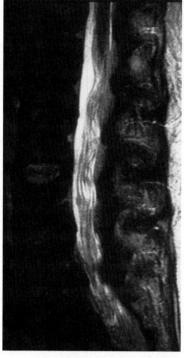

FIGURE 65.2

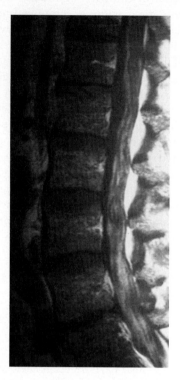

FIGURE 65.3

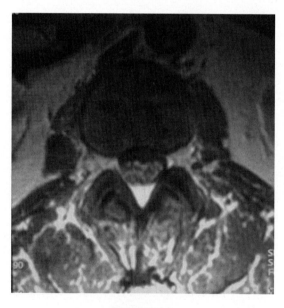

FIGURE 65.4

HISTORY

A 60-year-old with multiple myeloma, now with paresthesias.

FINDINGS

Sagittal T1-weighted image without contrast (Fig. 65.1) shows diffuse abnormal mottled signal intensity from all the vertebral bodies. There is abnormal, slightly increased signal intensity involving the caudal thecal sac and clumping of the cauda equina. T2-weighted image (Fig. 65.2) windowed for better visualization of the cauda equina shows prominence diffusely of the roots that appears clumped. The sagittal and axial (Figs. 65.3 and 65.4) T1-weighted images following contrast material show marked and diffuse enhancement along the cauda equina. There is also patchy enhancement of the vertebral bodies.

DIAGNOSIS

Myelomatous meningitis.

DISCUSSION

Patients with aggressive myeloma may develop myelomatous meningitis with extensive plasma cell infiltration of the meninges and a CSF pleocytosis. If the meninges are invaded by myeloma cells as well as being present along the leptomeninges, the CSF protein concentration will become elevated, and myeloma cells will be present in the CSF. MR findings show a combination of myelomatous vertebral body change with low signal on T1-weighted images, and changes of leptomeningeal disease. The leptomeningeal disease is identified by clumping of the roots and contrast enhancement of the leptomeninges.

BIBLIOGRAPHY

Camacho J, Arnalich F, Anciones B, et al. The spectrum of neurological manifestations in myeloma. *J Med* 1985;16:597–611.

Quint DJ, Levy R, Krauss JC. MR of myelomatous meningitis. *Am J Neuroradiol* 1995;16:1316–1317.

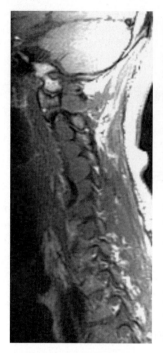

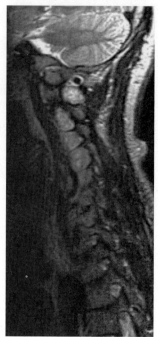

FIGURE 66.1   **FIGURE 66.2**

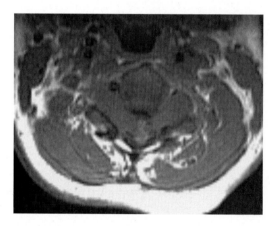

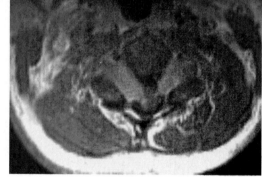

FIGURE 66.3   **FIGURE 66.4**

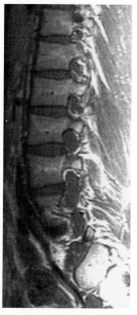

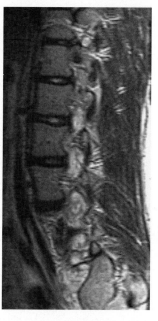

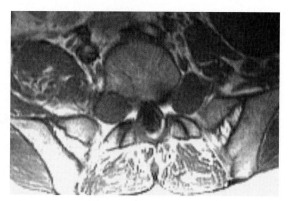

FIGURE 66.5   FIGURE 66.6   FIGURE 66.7

HISTORY

A 30-year-old with myelopathy.

FINDINGS

Sagittal T1-weighted image (Fig. 66.1) demonstrates a marked enlargement of multiple neural foramen by soft-tissue masses. The bony remodeling is smooth and consistent with a long-standing process. Sagittal T2-weighted image (Fig. 66.2) confirms the marked widening of multiple neural foramina with masses showing slight increased signal intensity. Axial T1-weighted images before (Fig. 66.3) and after (Fig. 66.4) contrast administration show symmetric soft-tissue masses with homogeneous enhancement that is both extradural and intradural. The combined masses show moderate cord effacement bilaterally. Sagittal T1-weighted image through the lumbar spine (Fig. 66.5) and the corresponding fast spin echo T2 image (Fig. 66.6) show multiple masses within the neuroforamina in the lumbar spine in the same patient. These lumbar masses are shown on the axial T1-weighted image (Fig. 66.7).

DIAGNOSIS

Neurofibromatosis, type I (NF-I).

DISCUSSION

Von Recklinghausen's disease (NF-I) is the most common phakomatosis and accounts for more than 90% of all cases of neurofibromatosis. It is an autosomal dominant disorder (like NF-II), although approximately 50% of cases arise by spontaneous mutation. The gene for NF-I has been linked to chromosome 17. It has three classic defining features: café au lait spots; peripheral cutaneous neurofibromas, which usually begin to appear at puberty; and Lisch nodules. Other neurologic manifestations include involvement of cranial nerves (CNs), the most common being the optic nerves and pathways in 15% to 35% (absent in other forms of NF), by pilocytic astrocytomas. Cranial nerves V (extracranial) and X and IX involvement is unusual. The other cranial nerves are rarely involved, with acoustic neuromas virtually nonexistent.

The NIH Consensus Development Conference established criteria for diagnosis of NF-I, which are to include two or more of the following:

1. Six or more café au lait spots greater than 5 mm in diameter in prepubertal and 15 mm in diameter in postpubertal patients;

2. Two or more neurofibromas of any type, or one plexiform neurofibroma;

3. Freckling in the axillary or inguinal regions;

4. Optic glioma;

5. Two or more Lisch nodules (pigmented iris hamartomas);

6. A distinctive osseous lesion, such as sphenoid dysplasia or thinning of long bone cortex, with or without pseudoarthrosis; and

7. A first-degree relative (sibling, parent, or child) with NF-I by the preceding criteria.

Primary involvement of the spinal cord is uncommon in NF-I, with cord compression by neurofibromas, vertebral collapse, and kyphoscoliosis more frequently seen. Intracranial or spinal arachnoid cysts are not uncommon, but meningiomas are very unusual. Peripheral nerve neurofibromas are generally extensive and may be gigantic plexiform tumors. These peripheral neurofibromas can be symptomatic, may be disfiguring, and may give rise to neurofibrosarcomas (5% to 10%). Schwannomas are much less frequent in NF-I than in NF-2.

BIBLIOGRAPHY

Egelhoff JC, Bates DJ, Ross JS, et al. Spinal MR findings in neurofibromatosis types 1 and 2. *Am J Neuroradiol* 1992;13:1071–1082.

Li MH, Holtas S. MR imaging of spinal neurofibromatosis. *Acta Radiol* 1991;32:279–285.

National Institutes of Health Consensus Development. Neurofibromatosis. *Arch Neurol* 1988;45:575–578.

Sze G, Abramson A, Krol G, et al. Gadolinium-DTPA in the evaluation of intradural extramedullary spinal disease. *Am J Roentgenol* 1988;150:911–921.

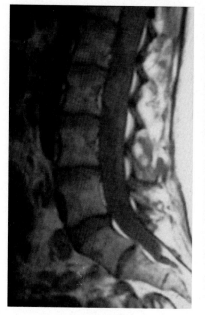

FIGURE 67.1   **FIGURE 67.2**

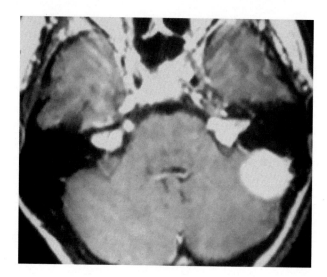

FIGURE 67.3

HISTORY

A 39-year-old with hearing loss.

FINDINGS

Sagittal T1-weighted images before (Fig. 67.1) and after (Fig. 67.2) contrast administration show multiple enhancing intradural masses. These are only vaguely identified on the study without contrast material. The vertebral bodies and posterior elements are otherwise normal in appearance. No mesodermal abnormalities are identified such as dural ectasia or posterior scalloping of the vertebral bodies. Axial T1-weighted image of the posterior fossa following contrast administration (Fig. 67.3) shows homogeneously enhancing masses involving both internal and auditory canals and extending into the cerebellopontine angle cisterns. Additionally, there is a homogeneously enhancing dural-based mass along the left lateral aspect of the left cerebellar hemisphere.

DIAGNOSIS

Neurofibromatosis, type II (NF-II).

DISCUSSION

The criteria for NF-II include (a) bilateral eighth-nerve masses or (b) NF-II in a first-degree relative and a unilateral eighth-nerve mass or one of the following: neurofibroma, meningioma, glioma, schwannoma, or juvenile posterior subcapsular lenticular opacity. NF-II is characterized by bilateral acoustic neurinomas in more than 90% of patients; few patients have cutaneous manifestations, whereas many have other tumors of the central nervous system, particularly meningiomas. Neurofibromas of and around the spine may be numerous, and intracranial and spinal meningiomas are frequent. Other features of NF-I are conspicuously absent in NF-II (e.g., Lisch nodules, optic pathway gliomas, segmental hypertrophy, pheochromocytomas, pseudoarthrosis, and other skeletal dysplasias). NF-II may not be obvious until the second or third decades or later and may be limited to acoustic neuromas without skin lesions. Cytogenetic work has shown an association with chromosome 22 in patients with NF-II. MR imaging findings in these are similar to those seen in patients with acoustic neuromas, intracranial and spinal meningiomas, or spinal neurofibromas. MR is the method of choice when an acoustic neuroma is suspected. It is also useful for detecting and determining the extent of the spinal, paraspinal, and retroperitoneal tumors.

The propensity for NF-II patients to have intramedullary ependymomas versus that of NF-I patients to have gliomas has been described by Egelhoff et al. They evaluated 28 neurofibromatosis type I (NF-I) patients and nine NF-II patients by MR. One NF-I patient had a biopsy-proven low-grade glioma; five NF-I patients had intradural, extramedullary masses; 16 NF-I patients had bony abnormalities. In the NF-II group, five patients demonstrated intramedullary masses (five/eight ependymomas) and nine patients had intradural, extramedullary masses (meningiomas, schwannomas). Eight out of 10 NF-I and four of nine NF-II patients had asymptomatic masses. Because of the propensity to develop significant asymptomatic as well as symptomatic intradural disease, screening of the entire spine with MR is recommended in both NF-I and NF-II patients.

BIBLIOGRAPHY

Egelhoff JC, Bates DJ, Ross JS, et al. Spinal MR findings in neurofibromatosis types 1 and 2. *Am J Neuroradiol* 1992;13:1071–1082.

National Institutes of Health Consensus Development. Neurofibromatosis. *Arch Neurol* 1988;45:575–578.

Sze G, Abramson A, Krol G, et al. Gadolinium-DTPA in the evaluation of intradural extramedullary spinal disease. *Am J Roentgenol* 1988;150:911–921.

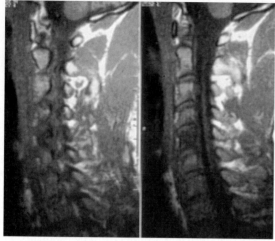

FIGURE 68.1

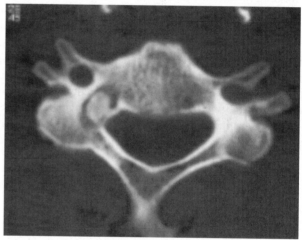

FIGURE 68.2

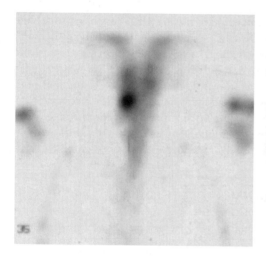

FIGURE 68.3

FIGURE 68.4

HISTORY

A 34-year-old with severe neck pain, worse at night.

FINDINGS

Sagittal T1-weighted images (Fig. 68.1) demonstrate abnormal low signal intensity within the C5 vertebral body. No epidural soft-tissue mass is seen. The posterior elements are normal. The abnormal signal within the C5 bodies is confirmed on the sagittal T2-weighted images (Fig. 68.2) which demonstrates high signal intensity. The remainder of the bodies are normal. The disk spaces adjacent to the C5 are normal as well.

Coronal SPECT study from a bone scan shows abnormal uptake involving the right side of the lower cervical vertebral bodies in the region of the MR marrow signal abnormality. The finding is further elucidated on the axial CT scan through the C5 body, which shows a bony nidus involving the right pedicle, with lucency surrounding it.

DIAGNOSIS

Osteoid osteoma.

DISCUSSION

Osteoid osteomas are approximately 10% of benign bone tumors. Most common spine locations are lumbar, followed by cervical and, less frequently, thoracic and sacral. They involve the posterior elements most commonly. Lesions classically present with pain and/or tenderness localized at the site of the lesion that is worse at night and can be relieved by aspirin. The pathology of these includes the multinucleated giant cells with a nidus consisting of vascular fibrous connective tissue surrounded by calcifying osteoid matrix. On MR, osteoid osteomas demonstrate a heterogeneous appearance. Calcification may show low signal on T1-weighted images but a halo of high signal on T2-weighted images as a result of inflammatory changes in the surrounding cancellous bone. CT shows small, rounded areas of low attenuation with or without calcification with sclerotic bone.

BIBLIOGRAPHY

Frassica FJ, Waltrip RL, Sponseller PD, et al. Clinicopathologic features and treatment of osteoid osteoma and osteoblastoma in children and adolescents. *Orthop Clin North Am* 1996;27:559–574.

Murphey MD, Andrews CL, Flemming DJ, et al. From the archives of the AFIP. Primary tumors of the spine: radiologic pathologic correlation. *Radiographics* 1996;5:1131–1158.

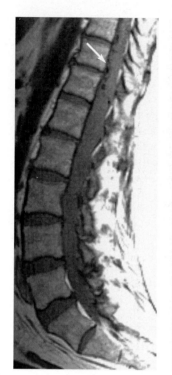

FIGURE 69.1

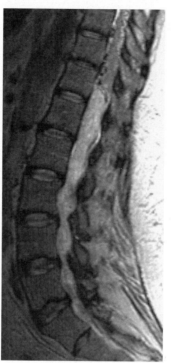

FIGURE 69.2

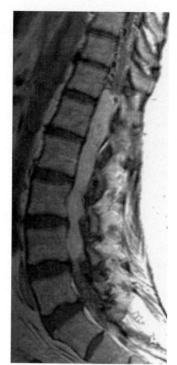

FIGURE 69.3

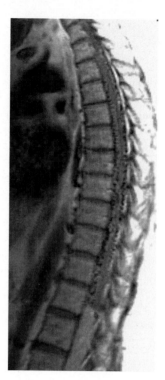

FIGURE 69.4

HISTORY

A 67-year-old with leg weakness.

FINDINGS

Sagittal T1-weighted image without contrast (Fig. 69.1) shows several serpentine flow voids involving the thoracolumbar junction anteriorly that appear intradural (*arrow*). There is abnormal increased signal from the CSF diffusely with no discrete mass identifiable. The sagittal T2-weighted fast spin echo sequence (Fig. 69.2) shows abnormal increased signal intensity throughout the thoracolumbar canal and confirms the abnormal flow void seen at the T11 level. Sagittal images of the lumbar (Fig. 69.3) and thoracic spine (Fig. 69.4) following contrast administration clearly define a discrete intradural and markedly enhancing mass extending inferiorly from the T12 level to the L4–5 level. Thoracic views show multiple serpentine flow voids consistent with multiple enlarged feeding vessels.

DIAGNOSIS

Paraganglioma.

DISCUSSION

Paragangliomas are neuroendocrine neoplasms that most often occur in relation to the adrenal gland. More than 90% of the extra adrenal paragangliomas are at the carotid body or glomus jugulare. However, these lesions can occur in a variety of unusual sites, such as intradurally. Other sites for paragangliomas within the CNS include pineal, petrous ridge, sella, and cauda equina. All reported cases of paragangliomas are intradural extramedullary lesions. Ages range between 13 and 70 years. These lesions do not produce any specific symptoms and behave like any other intradural extramedullary mass that may produce myelopathy, pain, or sciatica. Lesions are fairly nonspecific concerning signal intensity on MR and may show isointensity on T1- and moderate hyperintensity on T2-weighted images. The "salt and pepper" aspect that has been described with extra neural paragangliomas has not been described for intradural lesions. However, multiple feeding vessels can be visualized. These lesions tend to be misdiagnosed as ependymomas or schwannomas. They are highly vascular and tend to be encapsulated. No recurrence should be seen if they are completely excised. Growth is slow. Diagnosis is based on the typical light microscopic demonstration of neuroendocrine cells with a "Zellballen" pattern with argyrophil granules.

BIBLIOGRAPHY

Ashkenazi E, Onesti ST, Kader A, et al. Paraganglioma of the filum terminale: case report and literature review. *J Spinal Disord* 1998;11:540–542.

Boncoeur-Martel MP, Lesort A, Moreau JJ, et al. MRI of paraganglioma of the filum terminale. *J Comput Assist Tomogr* 1996;20:162–165.

Boukobza M, Foncin JF, Dowling-Carter D. Paraganglioma of the cauda equina: magnetic resonance imaging. *Neuroradiology* 1993;35:459–460.

Lamer S, Carlier RY, Parker F, et al. Paraganglioma of the cauda equina: MR findings. *J Neuroradiol* 1997;24:215–217.

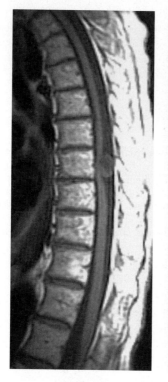

FIGURE 70.1

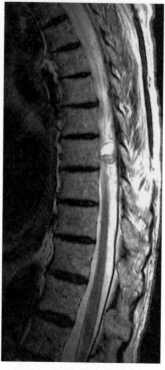

FIGURE 70.2

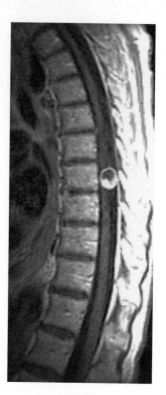

FIGURE 70.3

HISTORY

A 50-year-old with midthoracic pain and leg weakness.

FINDINGS

Sagittal T1-weighted image prior to contrast (Fig. 70.1) shows a discrete mass located dorsal to the midthoracic cord, which widens the CSF space on either side. The configuration is typical for an intradural extramedullary mass. The mass shows central cystic area that is high in signal intensity on the T2-weighted image (Fig. 70.2) surrounded by a more-solid-appearing low signal intensity. Following contrast administration (Fig. 70.3), there is peripheral enhancement surrounding the central cystic or necrotic area.

DIAGNOSIS

Schwannoma.

DISCUSSION

Not surprisingly, schwannomas are derived from Schwann cells. They typically involve the dorsal or sensory nerve roots and can be intradural, extradural, or both, forming a typical dumbbell configuration. Multiple schwannomas may occur in neurofibromatosis type II.

Schwannomas generally appear iso- to hypointense relative to spinal cord on T1-weighted images and increase signal intensity on T2-weighted images. Cyst formation can occur, showing more focal areas of high signal on T2 and diminished T1-weighted images. There can be variations in histology, with hemorrhage and collagen deposition that may predispose to even lower signal on T2-weighted images. Primary differentiating feature for these lesions is defining whether they are intramedullary or intradural and extramedullary. Once the intradural and extramedullary location has been defined using multiplanar imaging, the differential becomes relatively straightforward, including schwannoma, meningioma, and various leptomeningeal diseases (metastasis, granulomatous disease).

BIBLIOGRAPHY

Sevick RJ. Cervical spine tumors. *Neuroimaging Clin North Am* 1995;5:385–400.
Sze G, Abramson A, Krol G, et al. Gadolinium-DTPA in the evaluation of intradural extramedullary spinal disease. *Am J Roentgenol* 1988;150:911–921.

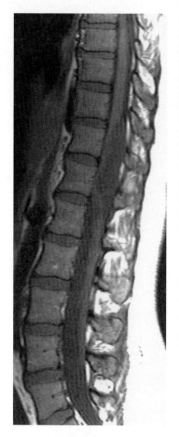
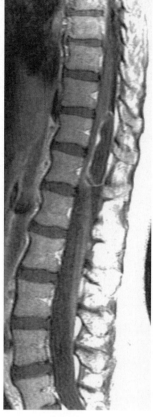
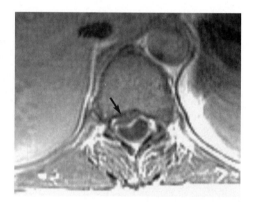

FIGURE 71.1   FIGURE 71.2   FIGURE 71.3

HISTORY

A 50-year-old with bladder/bowel dysfunction.

FINDINGS

Sagittal T1-weighted image (Fig. 71.1) demonstrates an ill-defined mass dorsal to the lower thoracic cord, which displaces the cord anteriorly. The lesion could either be intramedullary or intradural/extramedullary based on the unenhanced study. Following contrast material, the sagittal T1-weighted image (Fig. 71.2) shows peripheral enhance-ment of the lesion, with a more nodular component anteriorly. The lesion now looks more intradural/extramedullary in location. The intradural/extramedullary location is confirmed on the axial T1-weighted image following contrast administration, with the cord displaced anteriorly and to the right (*arrow*) (Fig. 71.3).

DIAGNOSIS

Schwannoma.

DISCUSSION

Schwannomas are lobulated soft-tissue masses composed fully of Schwann cells that arise eccentrically from peripheral sensory nerves. Schwannomas can arise *de novo* as solitary masses or can be seen in multiples with neurofibromatosis type II. Schwannomas tend to be more vascular than neuromas; both hemorrhage and cystic change are more common. Schwannomas generally vigorously enhance following contrast administration. These tumors mimic the appearance of meningiomas, showing a soft-tissue mass outlined by the low-signal-intensity CSF on T1 images, with displacement of the cord and highlighted CSF on T2 images. T2-weighted images typically show more high signal intensity than a typical meningioma. These tumors show prominent paramagnetic contrast enhancement. This can be homogeneous when the tumor is small and quite heterogeneous when the tumor is large. As with meningiomas, syringomyelic cavities can occur in the spinal cord secondary to the lesion compression.

BIBLIOGRAPHY

Sevick RJ. Cervical spine tumors. *Neuroimaging Clin North Am* 1995;5:385-400.
Sze G, Abramson A, Krol G, et al. Gadolinium-DTPA in the evaluation of intradural extramedullary spinal disease. *Am J Roentgenol* 1988;150:911–921.

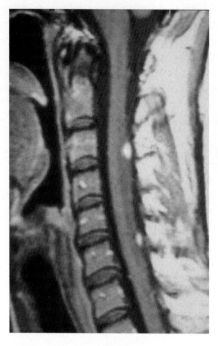

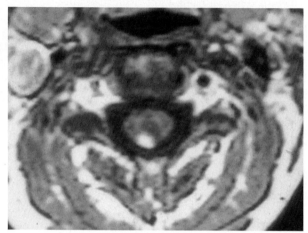

FIGURE 72.1

FIGURE 72.2

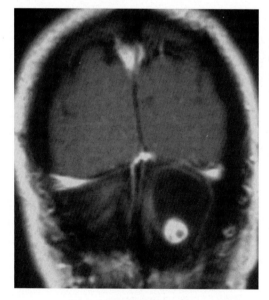

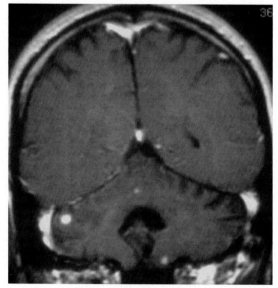

FIGURE 72.3

FIGURE 72.4

HISTORY

A 36-year-old with a history of renal mass.

FINDINGS

Sagittal (Fig. 72.1) and axial (Fig. 72.2) T1-weighted images following contrast administration show nodular areas of enhancement involving the dorsal aspect of the cervical cord, at the C3–4 and C5–6 levels. There is a mild enlargement of the cord at the C3–4 level. Two coronal T1-weighted images following contrast administration (Figs. 72.3 and 72.4) show multiple nodular areas of enhancement involving the cerebellar hemispheres. The largest enhancing nodular within the left hemisphere has a large associated cyst.

DIAGNOSIS

Hemangioblastomas in Von Hippel-Lindau syndrome.

DISCUSSION

Hemangioblastomas are rare, accounting for less than 2% of primary spinal tumors. They may involve the spinal cord or nerve roots, with 60% intramedullary and the remainder intradural/extramedullary in location. Most of these tumors occur as isolated lesions. However, they are often multiple, with one-third of cases associated with Von Hippel-Lindau syndrome. This autosomal dominant phakomatosis includes hemangioblastomas of the posterior fossa and cord, retinal angiomata, renal cell carcinoma, pheochromocytoma, and cysts or cystadenomas of the pancreas, adrenals, kidneys, and ovaries. Hemangioblastomas are histologically similar to angioblastic meningiomas and arise from the pia. They often present as intramedullary cysts with one or more vascular nodules. Approximately 40% are associated with expansion of the spinal cord, and dilated tortuous veins are characteristic. T1-weighted MR findings include an enlarged cord with predominantly hypointense area representing the cystic component that will become hyperintense on T2-weighted images. There can be extensive edema that widens the cord above and below the tumor nidus. These tumors will enhance vigorously with contrast because of their vascularity, helping to demarcate the high signal of the tumor from the surrounding edema. When a densely enhancing solid tumor nodule within a large "syrinx" cavity and associated "feeding" vessels is found in the cord, the examination should be continued into the cerebellum to exclude an additional hemangioblastoma.

BIBLIOGRAPHY

Choyke PL, Glenn GM, Walther MM, et al. Von Hippel-Lindau disease: genetic, clinical, and imaging features. *Radiology* 1995;194:629–642.

Friedman DP, Flanders AE, Tartaglino LM. Vascular neoplasms and malformations, ischemia, and hemorrhage affecting the spinal cord: MR imaging findings. *Am J Roentgenol* 1994;162:685–692.

Hoff DJ, Tampieri D, Just N. Imaging of spinal cord hemangioblastomas. *Can Assoc Radiol J* 1993;44:377–383.

Sze G, Krol G, Zimmerman RD, et al. Intramedullary disease of the spine: diagnosis using gadolinium-DTPA-enhanced MR imaging. *Am J Roentgenol* 1988;151:1193–1204.

CASE 73

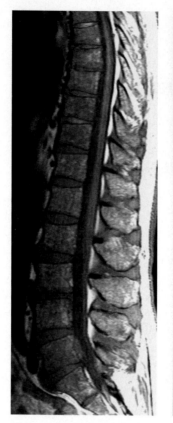

FIGURE 73.1

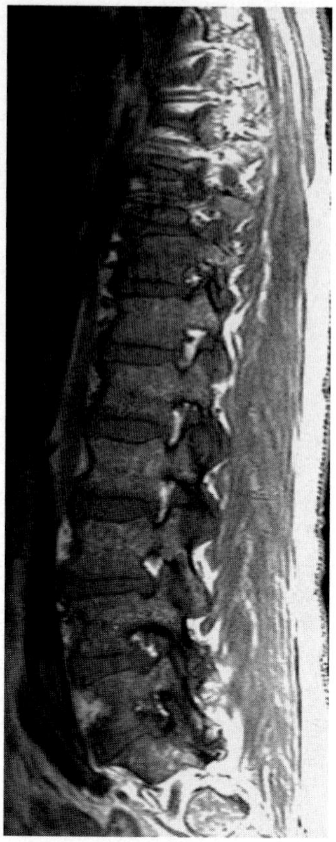

FIGURE 73.2

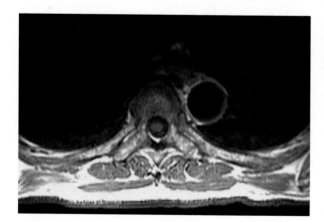

FIGURE 73.3

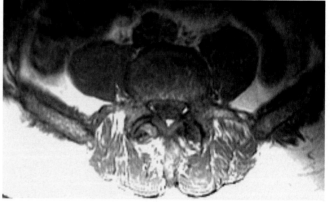

FIGURE 73.4

HISTORY

A 77-year-old with back pain and right leg pain. Plain films show a focal lytic right femoral lesion.

FINDINGS

Two sagittal T1-weighted images through the thoracolumbar spine (Figs. 73.1 and 73.2) demonstrate a diffuse mottled or speckled pattern of the marrow throughout all the vertebral bodies and posterior elements. The diffuse nature of the bone abnormality is confirmed on the thoracic axial T1-weighted (Fig. 73.3) and the lumbar axial at the L5–S1 level (Fig. 73.4). There is mottled signal intensity from the ribs, posterior elements, and iliac wings.

DIAGNOSIS

Multiple myeloma.

DISCUSSION

Multiple myeloma is a progressive neoplastic proliferation of plasma cells resulting in marrow plasmacytosis, a monoclonal protein band at urine or serum electrophoresis. There are permeative or geographic lesions in the axial skeleton. Patients present with nonspecific constitutional symptoms, such as back pain, renal failure, or recurrent infections. Marrow involvement may take two forms, either diffuse infiltration or nodular deposits. On MR, T1-weighted images show diminished signal intensity that may also have a salt and pepper mixed pattern. Compression fractures are common.

BIBLIOGRAPHY

Libshitz HI, Malthouse SR, Cunningham D, et al. Multiple myeloma: appearance at MR imaging. *Radiology* 1992;182:833–837.

Ludwig H, Fruhwald F, Tscholakoff D, et al. Magnetic resonance imaging of the spine in multiple myeloma. *Lancet* 1987;2:364–366.

Murphey MD, Andrews CL, Flemming DJ, et al. From the archives of the AFIP. Primary tumors of the spine: radiologic pathologic correlation. *Radiographics* 1996;16:1131–1158.

Rahmouni A, Divine M, Mathieu D, et al. Detection of multiple myeloma involving the spine: efficacy of fat-suppression and contrast-enhanced MR imaging. *Am J Roentgenol* 1993;160:1049–1052.

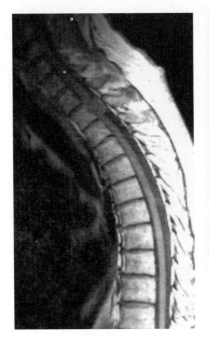

FIGURE 74.1

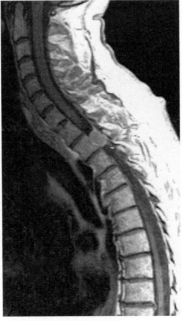

FIGURE 74.2

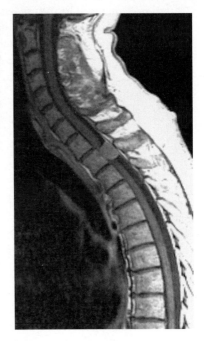

FIGURE 74.3

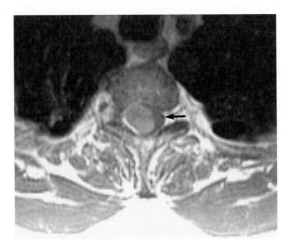

FIGURE 74.4

HISTORY

A 55-year-old with leg weakness and paresthesias.

FINDINGS

The unenhanced sagittal T1-weighted image (Fig. 74.1) shows a well-defined lesion at the cervical thoracic junction that appears to displace the cord anteriorly. Following contrast administration, two sagittal T1-weighted images (Figs.

74.2 and 74.3) better define the homogeneous mass, which has a dural base posteriorly. The mass displaces the cord anteriorly and is clearly intradural/extramedullary. The degree of mass effect upon the cord is better defined on the axial

T1-weighted image following contrast (Fig. 74.4). The cord is displaced and compressed to the left within the thecal sac (*arrow*), with the remainder of the sac containing the intradural mass, which shows diffuse enhancement.

DIAGNOSIS

Meningioma.

DISCUSSION

The typical patient with intradural/extramedullary meningioma is female and more than 40 years of age. Eighty percent of the lesions are found in the thoracic spine. Meningiomas are the most common tumor of the foramen magnum. Rarely, they can be both intradural and extradural. They may also be multiple. There are four histologic types of meningiomas: meningothelial, fibroblastic, psammomatous, and angiomatous. Meningiomas are calcified in more than 70% of cases. Sagittal and axial T1-weighted images show a small soft-tissue mass in the canal that is isointense to the spinal cord and will displace it. T2-weighted images show the tumors as low signal intensity surrounded by high-signal-intensity CSF. Typically, these uniformly and intensely enhance following contrast administration. There may be a cystic syrinx in the adjacent spinal cord secondary to compression and local CSF flow derangement.

BIBLIOGRAPHY

Roux FX, Nataf F, Pinaudeau M, et al. Intraspinal meningiomas: review of 54 cases with discussion of poor prognosis factors and modern therapeutic management. *Surg Neurol* 1996;46:458–463.

Sevick RJ. Cervical spine tumors. *Neuroimaging Clin North Am* 1995;5:385–400.

Sze G, Abramson A, Krol G, et al. Gadolinium-DTPA in the evaluation of intradural extramedullary spinal disease. *Am J Roentgenol* 1988;150:911–921.

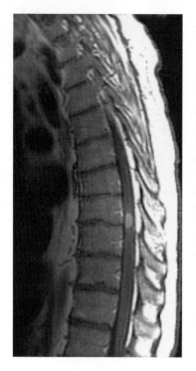

FIGURE 75.1

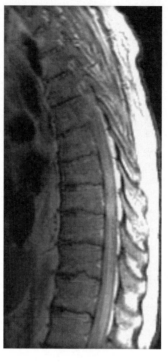

FIGURE 75.2

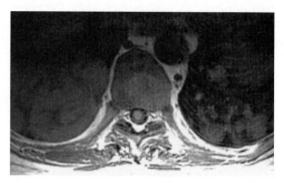

FIGURE 75.3

HISTORY

A 50-year-old with lung nodules and new-onset myelopathy.

FINDINGS

Sagittal T1-weighted image following contrast administration (Fig. 75.1) shows a focal area of enhancement within the midthoracic cord. No additional lesions are identified. The cord shows high signal intensity on the sagittal spin-density-weighted image (Fig. 75.2). The enhancing nidus within the cord is also shown on the axial T1-weighted image following contrast material (Fig. 75.3). Multiple lesions also present within the lung base, particularly on the left.

DIAGNOSIS

Cord metastasis from renal cell carcinoma.

DISCUSSION

Intramedullary cord metastases are considered rare but may be increasing in visualization with the wide availability of MR. In autopsy studies where the spinal cord is examined routinely, they comprise nearly 4% of the metastatic tumors affecting the spinal cord, with an overall prevalence of at least 1% in patients who die with cancer. Prolonged cancer survival has produced an increase in the incidence of CNS metastases in the natural history of some cancers. This has been clearly demonstrated in hematologic malignancies and in small cell carcinoma of the lung. The spinal cord could provide a sanctuary for such tumors because the blood-brain barrier is impermeable to most systemic chemotherapeutic agents. The most common sources of cord metastases include lung, breast, melanoma, lymphoma, and kidney. In 50% of these cases the primary tumor is the lung. Clinical presentations vary considerably, but mainly include pain, either local or radicular. The pain may develop suddenly in association with exertion, cough or back injury. Percussion tenderness, straight leg raise pain, and pain with straining or deep inspiration are not uncommon symptoms. Weakness, hemiparesis or paraparesis can occur.

BIBLIOGRAPHY

Dunne JW, Harper CG, Pamphlett R. Intramedullary spinal cord metastases: A clinical and pathological study of nine cases. *Q J Med* 1986;61:1003–1020.

Sze G, Krol G, Zimmerman RD, et al. Intramedullary disease of the spine: diagnosis using gadolinium-DTPA-enhanced MR imaging. *Am J Roentgenol* 1988;151:1193–1204.

Tognetti F, Lanzino G, Calbucci F. Metastases of the spinal cord from remote neoplasms: study of five cases. *Surg Neurol* 1988;30:220–227.

Winkelman MD, Adelstein DJ, Karlins NL. Intramedullary spinal cord metastasis: diagnostic and therapeutic considerations. *Arch Neurol* 1987;44:526–531.

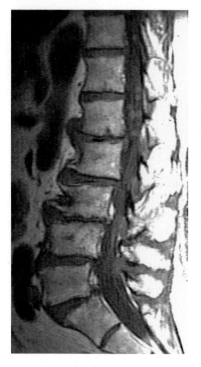

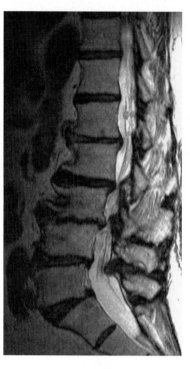

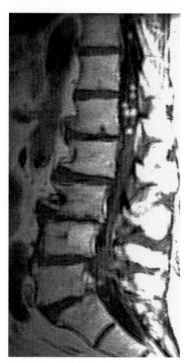

FIGURE 76.1   FIGURE 76.2   FIGURE 76.3

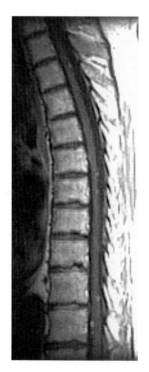

FIGURE 76.4

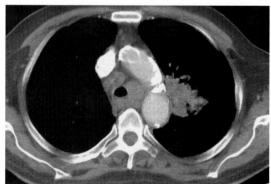

FIGURE 76.5

HISTORY

A 55-year-old with lung carcinoma, now with leg pain.

FINDINGS

Sagittal T1-weighted image without contrast (Fig. 76.1) demonstrates multiple well-defined nodular areas of increased signal intensity within the thecal sac and along the course of the cauda equina, particularly at the L1 level. Sagittal T2-weighted image (Fig. 76.2) confirms the abnormal intradural nodular lesions seen at the L1 level. There is incidental diffuse degenerative disk disease. Following contrast administration, the sagittal T1-weighted image (Fig. 76.3) shows multiple enhancing intradural lesions studding the cauda equina. Additional lesions are seen intradurally at the L5 level. The multiplicity of lesions is further confirmed on the sagittal T1-weighted image of the thoracic spine (Fig. 76.4). The axial CT section through the chest following contrast administration shows a left lung mass (Fig. 76.5) as well as mediastinal lymphadenopathy.

DIAGNOSIS

Leptomeningeal metastasis.

DISCUSSION

Leptomeningeal tumors are only adequately depicted with the use of contrast material. The difficulty in recognizing leptomeningeal disease on unenhanced images may be related to (a) the manner in which leptomeningeal metastases spread along the nerve root sleeves without forming discrete masses and (b) the signal characteristics of these lesions, which may be close to those of the surrounding CSF. Partial volume averaging can also be a problem with very small nodules of tumor surrounded by CSF. Motion artifacts and CSF pulsations may also contribute to inadequate visualization of small-drop metastases. In a study of patients with documented intradural/extramedullary disease, Sze showed that contrast greatly enhanced intradural/extramedullary nodules as small as 2 to 3 mm in diameter and thus showed leptomeningeal spread of tumor. Marked contrast enhancement was present in nine of 12 patients; milder enhancement, in one patient; equivocal enhancement, in one; and no enhancement in one. Not only were small lesions easily visualized following contrast administration, but leptomeningeal disease was more readily recognized in several patients than on CT myelography.

The list of tumors that may seed the CSF is long, but the main offenders are cranial ependymomas, glioblastomas, and medulloblastomas (especially in the pediatric population). Additional malignancies that can spread less commonly are ependymoma, pineoblastoma, germinoma, retinoblastoma, and choroid-plexus carcinoma. Lesions outside the CNS that are capable of spreading along the leptomeninges include carcinoma of the lung and breast as well as lymphoma, leukemia, and melanoma. Clinical presentation tends to be nonspecific and may include neck or back pain, with occasional focal deficits, including cranial nerve palsies and sphincter or motor dysfunction. CSF cytology is necessary for diagnosis. T2 imaging may be unrevealing. Administration of contrast material with T1-weighted images demonstrates a linear and nodular enhancement pattern along the leptomeninges. It must be remembered that the overall sensitivity of unenhanced and enhanced MR examinations is low in patients with proven histologic evidence of neoplastic seeding, so examination of the CSF remains the gold standard.

BIBLIOGRAPHY

DeAngelis LM. Current diagnosis and treatment of leptomeningeal metastasis. *J Neurooncol* 1998;38:245–252.

Sugahara T, Korogi Y, Hirai T, et al. Contrast-enhanced T1-weighted three-dimensional gradient-echo MR imaging of the whole spine for intradural tumor dissemination. *Am J Neuroradiol* 1998;19:1773–1779.

Sze G. Advancing techniques in spinal MR imaging: but are they necessary for spinal leptomeningeal tumor? *Am J Neuroradiol* 1998;19:1595–1596.

Sze G, Abramson A, Krol G, et al. Gadolinium-DTPA in the evaluation of intradural extramedullary spinal disease. *Am J Roentgenol* 1988;150:911–921.

Yousem DM, Patrone PM, Grossman RI. Leptomeningeal metastases: MR evaluation. *J Comput Assist Tomogr* 1990;14:255–261.

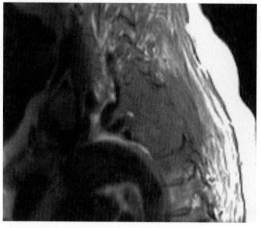

FIGURE 77.1

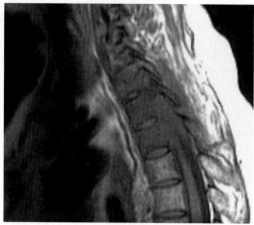

FIGURE 77.2

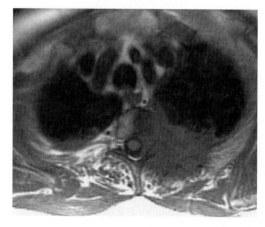

FIGURE 77.3

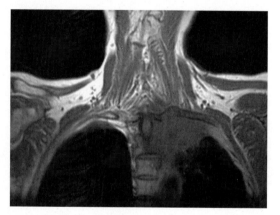

FIGURE 77.4

HISTORY

A 53-year-old with left arm pain, being evaluated for cervical disk disease.

FINDINGS

Sagittal T1-weighted images in the left parasagittal region (Figs. 77.1 and 77.2) show abnormally low signal intensity involving the cervicothoracic vertebral bodies with extension into the adjacent soft tissues and lung apex as well as posteriorly, where the facets are involved. Axial T1-weighted image (Fig. 77.3) also shows the mass involving the vertebral bodies, left paravertebral region, lung apex, and posterior areas, with extension into the soft tissues and laminae dorsally. The coronal T1-weighted image (Fig. 77.4) better defines the relationship of the apical mass, with the vertebral body and rib involvement.

DIAGNOSIS

Superior sulcus tumor.

DISCUSSION

Pancoast's tumors, or superior sulcus tumors, are apical lung tumors at the superior thoracic inlet that can produce a constellation of characteristic symptoms and signs called Pancoast's syndrome. These include shoulder and arm pain along the distribution of the eight cervical trunks and first and second thoracic nerves, Horner's syndrome, and weakness and atrophy of the muscles of the hand. Most cases of Pancoast's syndrome are caused by non–small-cell bronchogenic carcinomas, followed by adenocarcinoma and large-cell carcinoma. The clinical differential would include other primary thoracic neoplasms, metastases, infection, neurogenic thoracic outlet syndromes, and pulmonary amyloid nodules. CT and MR are the mainstays for imaging of these lesions. MR better appreciates chest wall invasion and is superior to CT with respect to tumor extension into the brachial plexus and vascular structures. Treatment is by en bloc resection of the tumor and chest wall, which may be accompanied by resection of involved paravertebral sympathic chain, lower trunks of the brachial plexus, and in some cases, subclavian artery and thoracic vertebrae. Tumor resection is also performed by lobectomy. Follow-up is by radiotherapy, which can also be used as a primary treatment modality. Palliation is achieved in 90% of these patients. Overall 5-year survival after combined preoperative radiotherapy and extended surgical resection is around 35%.

BIBLIOGRAPHY

Arcasoy SM, Jett JR. Superior pulmonary sulcus tumors and Pancoast's syndrome. *N Engl J Med* 1997;337:1370–1376.
Attar S, Krasna MJ, Sonett JR, et al. Superior sulcus (Pancoast) tumor: experience with 105 patients. *Ann Thorac Surg* 1998;66:193–198.
Laissy JP, Soyer P, Sekkal SR, et al. Assessment of vascular involvement with magnetic resonance angiography (MRA) in Pancoast syndrome. *Magn Reson Imaging* 1995;13:523–530.

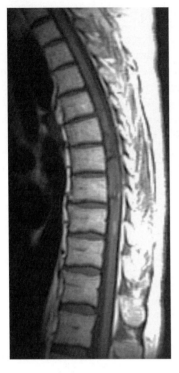

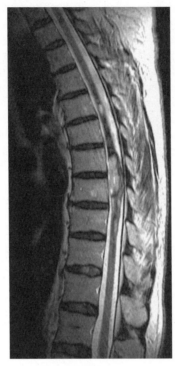

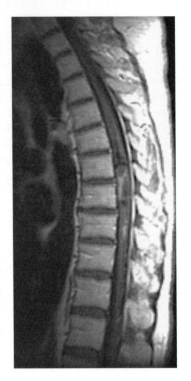

FIGURE 78.1

FIGURE 78.2

FIGURE 78.3

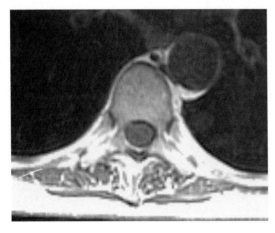

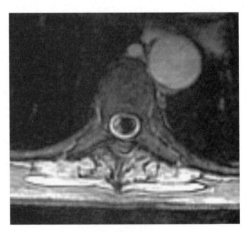

FIGURE 78.4

FIGURE 78.5

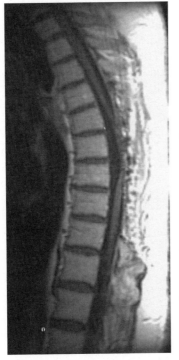
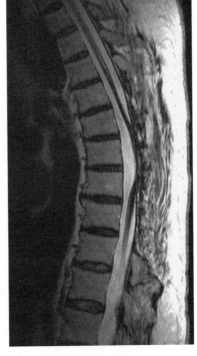

FIGURE 78.6   **FIGURE 78.7**

HISTORY

A 53-year-old with myelopathy.

FINDINGS

Sagittal T1-weighted image of the thoracic spine (Fig. 78.1) shows a fusiform enlargement of midthoracic cord with heterogeneous signal intensity within it. Linear areas of quite low signal intensity appear to cap the lesion centrally. More punctate and linear areas of high signal intensity are seen above and below the lesion, consistent with hemorrhage. The sagittal T2-weighted image (Fig. 78.2) also shows the heterogeneous nature of the lesion with the fusiform enlargement. Low signal intensity is seen within the upper segment of the thoracic cord, reflecting either hemorrhage or hemosiderin deposition. Sagittal T1-weighted image following contrast administration (Fig. 78.3) shows mild enhancement within the lesion and outlines the hemosiderin capping. Axial T1-weighted image without contrast (Fig. 78.4) and axial gradient echo image (Fig. 78.5) show the hemosiderin staining of the lesion itself. Following surgery, the sagittal T1-weighted image (Fig. 78.6) and sagittal fast spin echo T2-weighted image (Fig. 78.7) show local tethering of the cord to the operative site but no evidence of a discrete mass. There is diffuse hemosiderin staining of a long segment of the cord.

DIAGNOSIS

Thoracic ependymoma.

DISCUSSION

Ependymomas can involve any portion of the spinal cord, but they particularly affect the conus and filum terminale. Myxopapillary subtype is particularly common. Ependymomas typically present in the fourth to fifth decade of life, typically with complaints of back pain. Prognosis following surgery and radiation therapy can be quite good. On MR, ependymomas appear as a fusiform enlargement of the cord, or as lobulated extramedullary mass involving the filum terminale and cauda equina. These lesions may appear much like astrocytomas, being relatively diminished on T1-weighted images and increased on T2-weighted images. Contrast enhancement can be variable. Nearly half of ependymomas may be associated with cystic cavities within the cord. Ependymomas also classically are associated with evidence of old hemorrhage, showing hemosiderin or ferritin deposition with the typical susceptibility effects on T2* gradient echo images. This patient did well following surgery (despite the atrophy, tethering, and hemosiderin staining of the thoracic cord) and could ambulate with a walker.

BIBLIOGRAPHY

Bourgouin PM, Lesage J, Fontaine S, et al. A pattern approach to the differential diagnosis of intramedullary spinal cord lesions on MR imaging. *Am J Roentgenol* 1998;170:1645–1649.

Fine MJ, Kricheff II, Freed D, et al. Spinal cord ependymomas: MR imaging features. *Radiology* 1995;197:655–658.

Kahan H, Sklar EM, Post MJ, et al. MR characteristics of histopathologic subtypes of spinal ependymoma. *Am J Neuroradiol* 1996;17:143–150.

Lefton DR, Pinto RS, Martin SW. MRI features of intracranial and spinal ependymomas. *Pediatr Neurosurg* 1998;28:97–105.

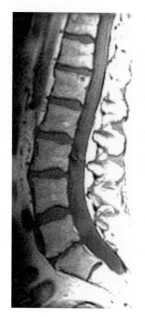

FIGURE 79.1

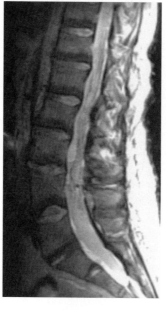

FIGURE 79.2

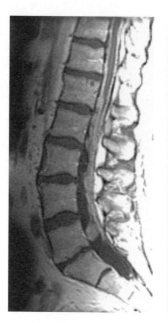

FIGURE 79.3

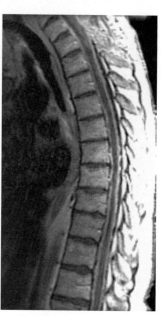

FIGURE 79.4

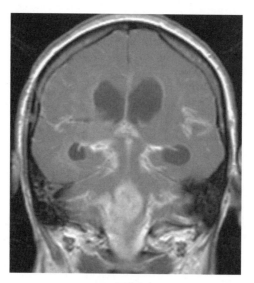

FIGURE 79.5

HISTORY

A 71-year-old with lung carcinoma, now with leg pain and weakness.

FINDINGS

Sagittal T1-weighted image without contrast (Fig. 79.1) shows ill-defined increased signal intensity throughout the thecal sac, with a poorly defined cauda equina and conus.

Sagittal T2-weighted image (Fig. 79.2) continues to show abnormal signal intensity throughout the thecal sac and apparent clumping of the cauda equina. Following contrast administration, sagittal T1-weighted image (Fig. 79.3) outlines diffuse abnormal leptomeningeal enhancement, coating the distal thoracic cord and cauda equina with both linear and modular patterns. Sagittal T1-weighted image to the thoracic spine (Fig. 79.4) also shows the diffuse leptomeningeal enhancement outlining the cord, seen as central low signal intensity. Coronal T1-weighted image of the brain (Fig. 79.5) following contrast administration shows diffuse abnormal leptomeningeal enhancement, particularly centered about the fourth ventricle.

DIAGNOSIS

Leptomeningeal metastasis.

DISCUSSION

The list of tumors that may seed the CSF is long, but the main offenders are cranial ependymomas, glioblastomas, and PNETs (primitive neuroectodermal tumors—i.e., medulloblastomas). Additional malignancies that can spread less commonly are pineoblastoma, germinoma, retinoblastoma, and choroid-plexus carcinoma. Lesions outside the CNS that are capable of spreading along the leptomeninges include carcinoma of the lung and breast, as well as lymphoma, leukemia, and melanoma. Clinical presentation tends to be nonspecific and may include neck or back pain, with occasional focal deficits, including cranial nerve palsies as well as sphincter or motor dysfunction. CSF cytology is necessary for diagnosis. T2 imaging may be unrevealing. Administration of contrast material with T1-weighted images demonstrates a linear and nodular enhancement pattern along the leptomeninges. The MR-enhanced study (sagittal survey scan over a large segment of the spine supplemented by axial scans) is more sensitive than myelography followed by CT. The overall sensitivity of unenhanced and enhanced MR examinations is low in patients with proven histologic evidence of neoplastic seeding, so examination of the CSF remains the gold standard. Thirty percent of patients with negative imaging studies will have a positive CSF study.

BIBLIOGRAPHY

DeAngelis LM. Current diagnosis and treatment of leptomeningeal metastasis. *J Neurooncol* 1998;38:245–252.

Sugahara T, Korogi Y, Hirai T, et al. Contrast-enhanced T1-weighted three-dimensional gradient-echo MR imaging of the whole spine for intradural tumor dissemination. *Am J Neuroradiol* 1998;19:1773–1779.

Sze GK. Advancing techniques in spinal MR imaging: but are they necessary for spinal leptomeningeal tumor? *Am J Neuroradiol* 1998;19:1595–1596.

Sze G, Abramson A, Krol G, et al. Gadolinium-DTPA in the evaluation of intradural extramedullary spinal disease. *Am J Roentgenol* 1988;150:911–921.

Yousem DM, Patrone PM, Grossman RI. Leptomeningeal metastases: MR evaluation. *J Comput Assist Tomogr* 1990;14:255–261.

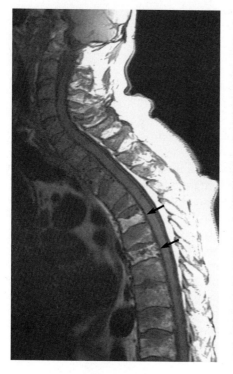

FIGURE 80.1

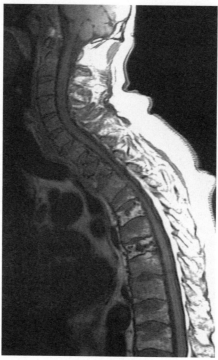

FIGURE 80.2

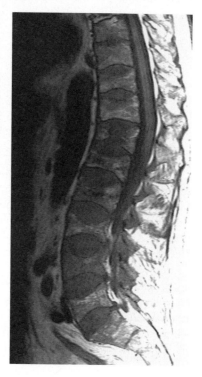

FIGURE 80.3

HISTORY

A 67-year-old with back pain.

FINDINGS

Sagittal T1-weighted images to the cervicothoracic spine (Fig. 80.1, 2) and through the thoracolumbar spine (Fig. 80.3) demonstrate multiple compression fractures through nearly all the thoracic and lumbar vertebral bodies. There is a diffuse speckled or mottled pattern of signal intensity throughout all the visualized vertebral bodies. Additionally, the T5 and T7 bodies show a more speckled or heterogeneous pattern with central areas of low signal intensity, with other areas of higher signal intensity reflecting fatty marrow infiltration (*arrows*).

DIAGNOSIS

Multiple myeloma following vertebroplasty.

DISCUSSION

Multiple myeloma is a malignancy of plasma cells affecting the bone marrow. It is associated with a monoclonal immunoglobulin in the blood and/or urine. The clinical staging system by Durie and Salmon that is often used follows.

Stage I consists of all of the following:
1. Hemoglobin value >100 g/L;
2. Serum calcium value normal;
3. Normal plain films'
4. Low M-component production rates.

Stage II consists of what is not stage I or stage III. Stage III includes one or more of the following:

1. Hemoglobin value <85 g/L;
2. Serum calcium value >12 mg/dL;
3. Lytic bone lesions;
4. High M-component production rates.

Stage I patients have low tumor burden of disease and do not usually require treatment until more aggressive disease occurs. Systemic therapy is beneficial in patients with stages II and III disease, with the greatest improvement in survival for stage III. Most patients who present with multiple myeloma do have stage III disease. The clinical pathology in myeloma relates to four main areas:

1. Myeloma cells within the bone marrow produces destruction of bone and hematopoietic abnormalities such as anemia, leukopenia, and thrombocytopenia.
2. Immune deficiencies lead to an increased susceptibility to infection.
3. The M-components are responsible for myeloma protein-related clinical manifestations such as the hyperviscosity, cryoglobulinemia, and amyloidosis.
4. Renal failure occurs secondary to the excretion of monoclonal light chains.

MR shows several patterns of marrow involvement. The marrow may be involved by focal nodular lesions with a background of normal high-signal-intensity fatty marrow. More diffuse involvement shows low signal intensity throughout the marrow. Patients with multiple myeloma may also show completely normal marrow by MR imaging. Patients with stage I disease with abnormal MR studies have more rapidly progressive disease than patients with normal marrow. With higher-grade disease, the spinal marrow pattern can be associated with clinical parameters of disease severity. Specifically, patients with stage III disease and a diffuse MR pattern have more severe abnormalities of hematologic parameters than those with a normal or focal pattern of disease. Response to initial induction chemotherapy has been shown to be better in patients with normal marrow MR than in those with focal or diffuse pattern, with stage III disease.

Vertebroplasty has become an important technique to stabilize the vertebral bodies in patients with myeloma who have compression fractures. This can produce dramatic decrease in pain. In this patient, the vertebral bodies that have been treated with vertebroplasty show a mixture of low signal intensity due to the methylmethacrylate utilized as well as an improved appearance of fatty high-signal-intensity marrow within the adjacent peripheral marrow.

BIBLIOGRAPHY

Cortet B, Cotten A, Boutry N, et al. Percutaneous vertebroplasty in patients with osteolytic metastases or multiple myeloma. *Rev Rhum Engl Ed* 1997;64:177–183.

Cotten A, Dewatre F, Cortet B, et al. Percutaneous vertebroplasty for osteolytic metastases and myeloma: effects of the percentage of lesion filling and the leakage of methyl methacrylate at clinical follow-up. *Radiology* 1996;200:525–530.

Deramond H, Depriester C, Galibert P, et al. Percutaneous vertebroplasty with polymethylmethacrylate: technique, indications, and results. *Radiol Clin North Am* 1998;36:533–546.

Durie BG, Salmon SE. A clinical staging system for multiple myeloma: correlation of measured myeloma cell mass with presenting clinical features, response to treatment, and survival. *Cancer* 1975;36:842–854.

Foerster J, Paraskeuas F. *Wintrobe's clinical hematology*, 10th ed. New York: Lippincott Williams & Wilkins, 1999:2650–2652.

Jensen ME, Evans AJ, Mathis JM, et al. Percutaneous polymethylmethacrylate vertebroplasty in the treatment of osteoporotic vertebral body compression fractures: technical aspects. *Am J Neuroradiol* 1997;18:1897–1904.

Lecouvet FE, Vende Berg BC, Michaux L, et al. Stage III multiple myeloma: clinical and prognostic value of spinal bone marrow MR imaging. *Radiology* 1998;209:653–660.

Libshitz HI, Malthouse SR, Cunningham D, et al. Multiple myeloma: appearance at MR imaging. *Radiology* 1992;182:833–837.

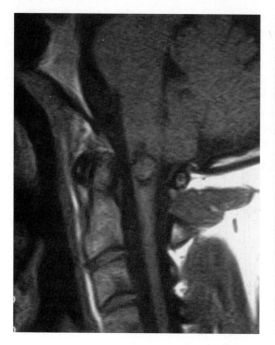

FIGURE 81.1

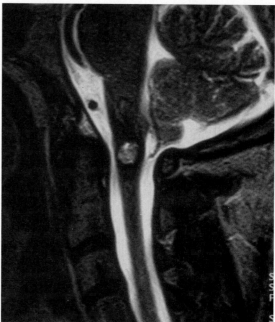

FIGURE 81.2

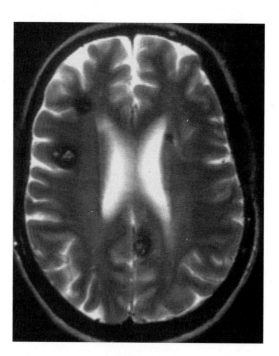

FIGURE 81.3

HISTORY

A 42-year-old with weakness and spasticity.

FINDINGS

Sagittal T1-weighted (Fig. 81.1) and fast spin echo T2-weighted (Fig. 81.2) images of the cervicomedullary junction show a heterogeneous mass involving the cervical cord at the C1 level. It shows peripheral low signal on both the T1- and T2-weighted images in mottled high and low signal intensity centrally. There is no evidence of edema surrounding the lesion. Axial T2-weighted spin echo image through the brain parenchyma (Fig. 81.3) shows multiple well-defined lesions and a speckled or mottled pattern. They are surrounded by low signal intensity rim and have no evidence of edema.

DIAGNOSIS

Cavernous angioma.

DISCUSSION

The MR appearance of a cryptic vascular malformation of the spinal cord is similar in appearance to the lesions in the brain. A nodular or punctate area of high signal on T1-weighted MR sequences represents the intraparenchymal core of subacute blood and chronic hemorrhage. This may be a "salt and pepper" pattern of mixed areas of high and low signal. The high signal from methemoglobin may persist for long periods of time. Low-intensity signal halo may be seen on all sequences, but especially T2-weighted spin echo and gradient echo images, due to hemosiderin deposition at the periphery of the bleed. Fast spin echo sequences tend to minimize this low signal due to susceptibility effects. As with all vascular malformations, the typical pattern is of little or no mass effect and no associated edema. Enhancement can be quite variable. With more recent hemorrhage, expansion of the cord can occur, which can produce cord edema. The diagnosis of a cryptic spinal malformation is supported by the presence of other, similar lesions elsewhere in the cord or brain. Up to 25% of such cryptic vascular malformations are multiple. Although malignant cord neoplasms may present as a hemorrhagic event, they usually expand the cord in a more irregular and less focal manner. In addition, abnormally high T2 signal due to edema is noticed distal to the epicenter of the bleed and the area. The incomplete halo of hemosiderin deposition that may signal a more aggressive lesion in the brain is generally not of much help in the cord.

BIBLIOGRAPHY

Acciarri N, Padovani R, Giulioni M, et al. Surgical treatment of spinal cavernous angiomas. *J Neurosurg Sci* 1993;37:209–215.

Duke BJ, Levy AS, Lillehei KO. Cavernous angiomas of the cauda equina: case report and review of the literature. *Surg Neurol* 1998;50:442–445.

Murphey MD, Fairbairn KJ, Parman LM, et al. From the archives of the AFIP. Musculoskeletal angiomatous lesions: radiologic-pathologic correlation. *Radiographics* 1995;15:893–917.

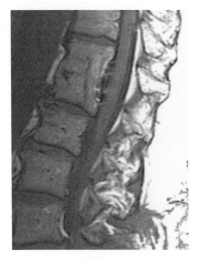
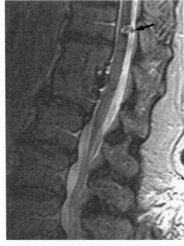
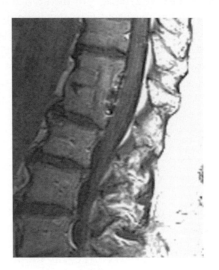

FIGURE 82.1   **FIGURE 82.2**   **FIGURE 82.3**

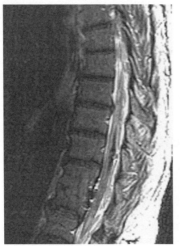
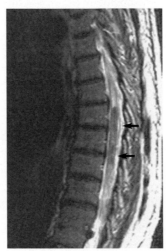

FIGURE 82.4   **FIGURE 82.5**

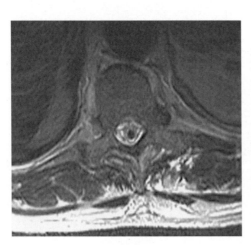
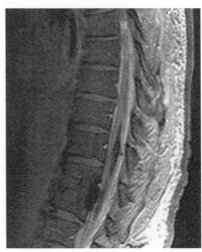

FIGURE 82.6   **FIGURE 82.7**

HISTORY

A 46-year-old patient who underwent lumbar laminectomy for disk disease, now with acute-onset paraplegia.

FINDINGS

Initial sagittal T1-weighted (Fig. 82.1) and sagittal fast spin echo T2-weighted (Fig. 82.2) images prior to the onset of paraplegia show postoperative fusion at T12 and L1, with metal artifacts seen within the anterior epidural space. The conus shows a focal area of heterogeneous signal intensity, particularly on the sagittal T2-weighted image along the dorsal aspect of the thoracic cord suspicious for small vascular malformation (*arrow*). At the time of onset of paraplegia 2 weeks later, the sagittal T1-weighted image (Fig. 82.3) shows mild enlargement of the thoracic cord but no other definite abnormality that is new. The sagittal T2-weighted images (Figs. 82.4 and 82.5) show abnormal low-signal-intensity narrowing extending more cephalad within the thoracic cord to the midthoracic level (*arrows*). The abnormal low signal is confirmed on both the axial gradient echo (Fig. 82.6) and the sagittal gradient echo images (Fig. 82.7).

DIAGNOSIS

Cord hemorrhage secondary to vascular malformation.

DISCUSSION

Hemorrhage within the cord can be caused by a variety of pathologies. The most common are trauma, spinal tumors, and arteriovenous malformations. Tumors in the region of the cauda equina and conus medullaris can cause parenchymal and even subarachnoid hemorrhage. The ependymoma is the most frequently encountered. The MR features of cord hemorrhage in the late acute and subacute stage will show the typical high signal intensity on T1-weighted images. Early on, as in this case, the T1-weighted images may not be helpful. If there is a concern of early hemorrhage, then it is mandatory to use either a T2-weighted sequence or, preferably, a gradient echo sequence. On these the early changes of deoxyhemoglobin will be seen as diminished signal intensity within the central aspect of the cord. Initial T1- and T2-weighted images in this patient show no evidence of hemorrhage. Instead a focal area of signal abnormality surrounded by low-signal-intensity hemosiderin on the T2-weighted images within the dorsal aspect of the lower thoracic cord reflects a small vascular malformation. Several weeks later, the patient presented with acute onset of paraplegia. Immediate imaging showed abnormal signal intensity within the substance of the cord, which "bloomed" on a gradient echo sequence. These findings are typical for an acute hemorrhage within the lower thoracic cord.

BIBLIOGRAPHY

Flanders AE, Spettell CM, Tartaglino LM, et al. Forecasting motor recovery after cervical spinal cord injury: value of MR imaging. *Radiology* 1996;201:649–655.

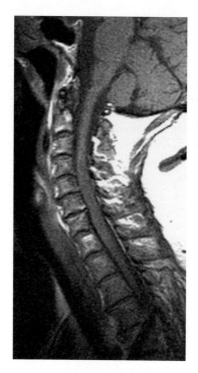

FIGURE 83.1

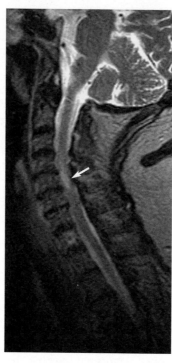

FIGURE 83.2

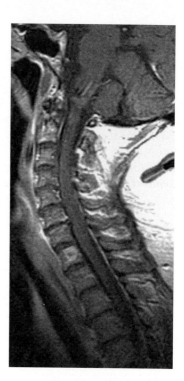

FIGURE 83.3

HISTORY

A 70-year-old now paraplegic after aortic aneurysm repair.

FINDINGS

Sagittal T1 image shows mild cord enlargement at the C5–7 levels (Fig. 83.1). There is mild diffuse cervical degenerative disease. Sagittal T2-weighted image (Fig. 83.2) shows focal abnormal increase signal intensity within the cervical cord at the C5 level (*arrow*). Following contrast administration, the sagittal T1-weighted image (Fig. 83.3) shows no abnormal intramedullary enhancement.

DIAGNOSIS

Cord infarct.

DISCUSSION

Most cases of spontaneous cord infarct occur in patients with thoracoabdominal aneurysms where the presumed mechanism is occlusion of the intercostal artery from which the anterior spinal artery rises. Dissecting aneurysms are associated with higher incidence of spinal cord ischemia. Other causes of infarction are many, such as hypotension, angiography, vertebral occlusion, dissection, trauma, and, rarely, disk herniation. Findings are fairly nonspecific, with the cord enlargement in increased T2-weighted images. Generally, there is no evidence of hemorrhage, and little enhancement. Signal abnormalities tend to involve the anterior horns of the gray matter, and as ischemia worsens, spreads posteriorly to involve the posterior horns. Yuh et al, stressed importance of findings outside the cord which could aid in their diagnosis. They looked at steps in the flow-void in the distal aorta caused by complete occlusion, and abnormal signal within the bone marrow due to vertebral body associated with vertebral body infarcts.

BIBLIOGRAPHY

Amano Y, Machida T, Kumazaki T. Spinal cord infarcts with contrast enhancement of the cauda equina: two cases. *Neuroradiology* 1998;40:669–672.

Faig J, Busse O, Salbeck R. Vertebral body infarction as a confirmatory sign of spinal cord ischemic stroke: report of three cases and review of the literature. *Stroke* 1998;29:239–243.

Haddad MC, Aabed al-Thagafi MY, Djurberg H. MRI of spinal cord and vertebral body infarction in the anterior spinal artery syndrome. *Neuroradiology* 1996;38:161–162.

Mascalchi M, Cosottini M, Ferrito G, et al. Posterior spinal artery infarct. *Am J Neuroradiol* 1998;19:361–363.

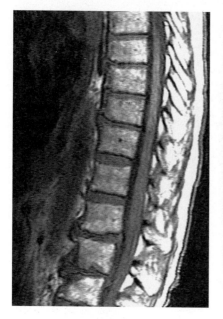

FIGURE 84.1

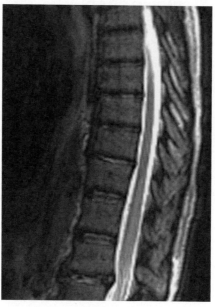

FIGURE 84.2

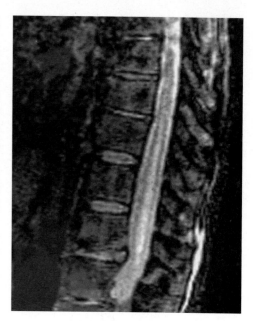

FIGURE 84.3

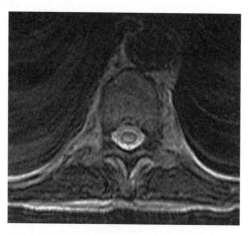

FIGURE 84.4

HISTORY

A 56-year-old with gastric carcinoma following celiac ganglion block, with acute-onset paraplegia.

FINDINGS

Sagittal T1-weighted image (Fig. 84.1) shows slight diminished signal intensity involving the distal thoracic cord and conus but with no other intradural lesions. Degenerative disease is seen at the thoracolumbar junction, with loss of disk space height and broad-based disk protrusions. The sagittal T2-weighted image (Fig. 84.2) demonstrates abnormal increased signal intensity involving the distal thoracic cord. The abnormal signal intensity is confirmed on the sagittal fast short inversion time inversion-recovery (STIR) image (Fig. 84.3) and the axial gradient echo sequence (Fig. 84.4).

DIAGNOSIS

Cord infarct.

DISCUSSION

The main arteries that comprise the spinal cord include the single anterior spinal artery and the paired posterior spinal arteries. These are contiguous along the longitudinal length of the cord. Contributions from radiculomedullary arteries occur at multiple levels, with the best known and largest being the artery of the Adamkiewicz. Cord infarction can be caused by a variety of abnormalities, particularly including embolic disease such as following aortic aneurysm repair. Hypotensive infarcts can occur in cardiac arrest. Other vascular abnormalities, such as vas-culitis and dissection, can occur. The MR findings are nonspecific but show high signal intensity on T2-weighted images. Cord enlargement can sometimes be seen on T1-weighted images. Contrast enhancement is not robust, but vague and patchy enhancement to a small degree may be seen after a few days following the infarct. Late changes show focal atrophy. The mechanism in this case may relate to extension of the neurolytic agent beyond the area of interest, with resultant direct neural and vascular damage.

BIBLIOGRAPHY

Brown E, Virapongse C, Gregorios JB. MR imaging of cervical spinal cord infarction. *J Comput Assist Tomogr* 1989;13:920–922.

Friedman DP, Flanders AE. Enhancement of gray matter in anterior spinal infarction. *Am J Neuroradiol* 1992;13:983–985.

Hirono H, Yamadori A, Komiyama M, et al. MRI of spontaneous spinal cord infarction: serial changes in gadolinium-DTPA enhancement. *Neuroradiology* 1992;34:95–97.

Takahashi S, Yamada T, Ishii K, et al. MRI of anterior spinal artery syndrome of the cervical spinal cord. *Neuroradiology* 1992;35:25–29.

Yuh WT, Marsh EE, Wang AK, et al. MR imaging of spinal cord and vertebral body infarction. *Am J Neuroradiol* 1992;13:145–154.

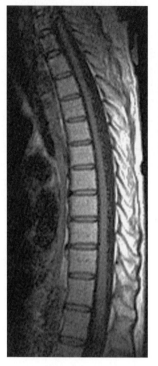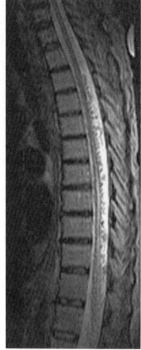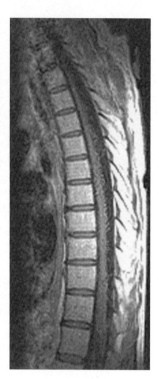

| FIGURE 85.1 | FIGURE 85.2 | FIGURE 85.3 |

HISTORY

A 60-year-old male with myelopathy.

FINDINGS

Sagittal T1-weighted image without contrast administration of the thoracic spine (Fig. 85.1) shows normal vertebral bodies and posterior elements. Thoracic cord is overall normal in size and signal intensity. There are multiple punctate foci of high and low signal intensity along the dorsal aspect of the thoracic cord. These punctate abnormali- ties are further demonstrated on the sagittal T2-weighted image (Fig. 85.2), which shows multiple small serpentine flow voids within the subarachnoid space dorsal to the thoracic cord. Following contrast administration (Fig. 85.3), the sagittal T1-weighted image shows mild patchy enhancement of these areas.

DIAGNOSIS

Dural fistula.

DISCUSSION

Spinal dural arteriovenous fistulas are also called dural malformations or radicular meningeal fistulas. These lesions are believed to be acquired and are particularly present in the thoracic and lower lumbar spine. Spinal dural arteriovenous fistulas are more common in men (3.4:1) more than 60 years of age. There is usually a considerable delay from symptom onset to time of diagnosis, averaging 27 months. Clinical findings include weakness, progressive clinical course, and myelopathy on examination. The nidus of the fistula is most often located between T6 and T12, and in the sacrum and intracranially in 8% to 9% each. Occurrence of sudden thrombophlebitis can produce rapid deterioration (most likely the cause of the Foix-Alajounine syndrome). Kendell and Logue in 1977 definitively defined the site of the arteriovenous shunting within the root sleeve. The symptoms are a product of intramedullary edema and ischemia secondary to raised venous backpressure within the varicose coronal veins. Gilbertson et al. have identified the high increased signal intensity on T2-weighted images within the cord as the most sensitive imaging finding in spinal dural fistula. However, flow voids were present in up to 45% of the cases. Contrast enhancement was common within the dilated vessels. Patchy intramedullary enhancement is also commonly seen and should not dissuade the physician from the diagnosis. MR angiography can be used to identify the fistula as well as its fistula site with either coronal or sagittal three-dimensional time-of-flight acquisitions following contrast administration. Willinsky et al. demonstrated that, following treatment of these fistulas, MR shows a resolution of enlarged subarachnoid vessels, cord enlargement, and hyperintensity on T2-weighted images. Nevertheless, the authors continue to recommend follow-up angiogram to be done in approximately 2 to 3 months following surgical or intervascular treatment, even in the face of supportive evidence of a more normal-appearing MR. Pathologic examination in dural fistula shows spinal cord changes identical to those described with nonhemorrhagic venous infarction of the spinal cord. This supports the conclusion that the myelopathy is mediated by venous hypertension, with changes including hyalinized vessels, arterialized veins, vascular calcification, and thrombosis.

BIBLIOGRAPHY

Bowen BC, Pattany PM. MR angiography of the spine. *Magn Reson Imaging Clin North Am* 1998;6:165–178.

Gilbertson JR, Miller GM, Goldman MS, et al. Spinal dural arteriovenous fistulas: MR and myelographic findings. *Am J Neuroradiol* 1995;16:2049–2057.

Kendall BE, Logue V. Spinal epidural angiomatous malformations draining into intrathecal veins. *Neuroradiology* 1977;13:181–189.

Larsson EM, Desai P, Hardin CW, et al. Venous infarction of the spinal cord resulting from dural arteriovenous fistula: MR imaging findings. *Am J Neuroradiol* 1991;12:739–743.

Masaryk T, Ross JS, Modic MT, et al. Radiculomeningeal vascular malformations of the spine: MR imaging. *Radiology* 1987;164:845–849.

Willinsky R, terBrugge K, Montanera W, et al. Posttreatment MR findings in spinal dural arteriovenous malformations. *Am J Neuroradiol* 1995;16(10): 2063–2071.

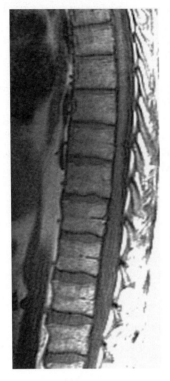

FIGURE 86.1

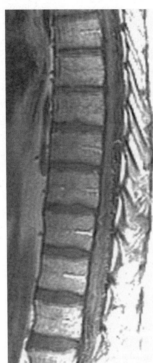

FIGURE 86.2

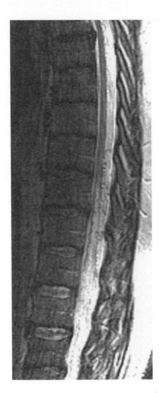

FIGURE 86.3

HISTORY

A 67-year-old with gradual-onset leg weakness.

FINDINGS

Sagittal T1-weighted image of the thoracolumbar junction (Fig. 86.1) shows mild prominence of the conus but no definite abnormality, with slightly diminished signal within the dorsal subarachnoid space. Following contrast administration, sagittal T1-weighted image (Fig. 86.2) shows diffuse serpentine abnormal enhancement along the cord surface both ventral and dorsal. This is confirmed on the sagittal fast spin echo T2-weighted image (Fig. 86.3). There are also abnormal increases in signal intensity within the distal thoracic cord and conus.

DIAGNOSIS

Dural fistula.

DISCUSSION

Dural vascular malformations are believed to be acquired lesions, typically presenting in the thoracic and thoracolumbar spine in patients over the age of 50. The mode of presentation is a slow, progressive myelopathy with lower-extremity paraparesis and bowel or bladder symptoms. Myelopathic symptoms are thought to be the product of intermedullary edema and ischemia related to raised intravenous pressure within the varicose and arterialized coronal veins around the spinal cord. Kendall and Logue described the dural site of arterial venous shunting in 1977. Successful treatment can either be achieved endovascularly or by simple ligation of the dominant intradural draining vessel. Imaging studies show low-signal dilated coronal veins in their expected peripheral and circumferential location about the spinal cord. Edema is seen within the cord as high signal on the T2-weighted images that relatively spares the periphery of the cord. This intramedullary signal abnormality can reverse following successful treatment. There may be patchy enhancement within the ischemic segment of the cord.

BIBLIOGRAPHY

Criscuolo GR, Rothbart D. Vascular malformations of the spinal cord: pathophysiology, diagnosis, and management. *Neurosurg Q* 1992;2:77–98.

Friedman DP, Flanders AE, Tartaglino LM. Vascular neoplasms and malformations, ischemia, and hemorrhage affecting the spinal cord: MR imaging findings. *Am J Roentgenol* 1994;162:685–692.

Kendall BE, Logue V. Spinal epidural angiomatous malformations draining into intrathecal veins. *Neuroradiology* 1997;13:181–189.

Lundqvist C, Berthelsen B, Sullivan M, et al. Spinal arteriovenous malformations: neurological aspects and results of embolization. *Acta Neurol Scand* 1990;82:51–58.

Masaryk TJ, Ross JS, Modic MT, et al. Radiculomeningeal vascular malformations of the spine: MR imaging. *Radiology* 1987;164:845–849.

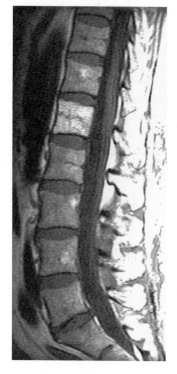

FIGURE 87.1

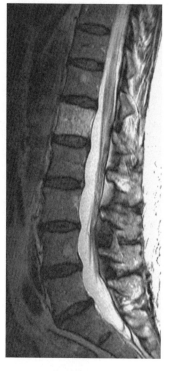

FIGURE 87.2

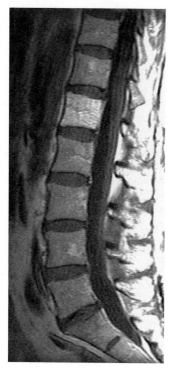

FIGURE 87.3

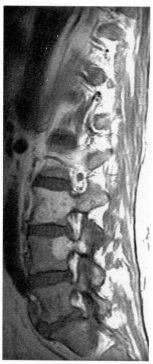

FIGURE 87.4

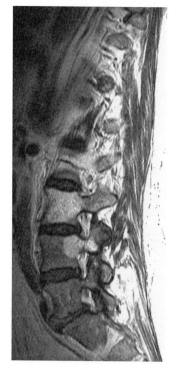

FIGURE 87.5

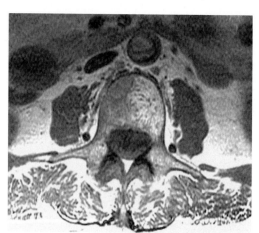

FIGURE 87.6

HISTORY

A 68-year-old being evaluated for metastatic disease.

FINDINGS

Sagittal T1-weighted image prior to contrast (Fig. 87.1) shows focal increased signal intensity within the L1 vertebral body with a slightly heterogeneous pattern. The sagittal fast spin echo T2-weighted image (Fig. 87.2) also shows high signal intensity that has a mottled or speckled pattern. Following contrast administration, the sagittal T1-weighted image (Fig. 87.3) shows no definite enhancement. No evidence of epidural extension is seen. Parasagittal T1-weighted image (Fig. 87.4) shows additional areas of high signal within the L4 and L3 bodies. At the L3 level, the high signal extends into the posterior elements. High signal is also seen on the parasagittal fast spin echo T2-weighted image (Fig. 87.5). Axial T1-weighted image without contrast (Fig. 87.6) better defines the mottled or corduroy pattern within the vertebral body.

DIAGNOSIS

Vertebral body hemangiomas.

DISCUSSION

Hemangiomas are slow-growing, benign lesions that have been demonstrated in 11% of spines at autopsy. These are rarely symptomatic. Most of these lesions are discovered incidentally. If they are symptomatic, they tend to occur in the thoracic region, presenting with pain and tenderness. Myelopathic symptoms may be attributable to pathologic fractures or vertebral body collapse, or epidural extension of tumor or epidural hematoma. Histologically, these are collections of thin-walled blood vessels or sinuses lined by endothelium that are interspersed among bony trabeculae and abundant adipose tissue. MR has a distinctive appearance, with modeled increased signal intensity due to the adipose tissue on T1-weighted images. Flow-related effects are not thought to contribute significantly to the MR appearance of these lesions, which also tend to follow fat on T2-weighted images but show more increased signal. Extradural components are more nonspecific in appearance, show isointensity to muscle, and do not show the high signal related to the abundant fat tissue.

BIBLIOGRAPHY

Fox MW, Onofrio BM. The natural history and management of symptomatic and asymptomatic vertebral hemangiomas. *J Neurosurg* 1993;78:36–45.
Ross JS, Masaryk TJ, Modic MT, et al. Vertebral hemangiomas: MR imaging. *Radiology* 1987;165:165–169.

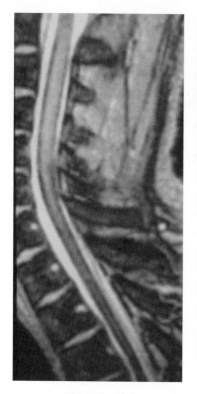

FIGURE 88.1

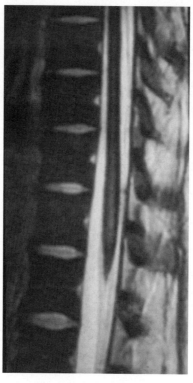

FIGURE 88.2

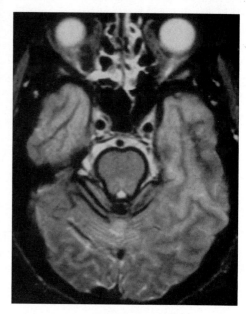

FIGURE 88.3

HISTORY

A 66-year-old with multiple cranial nerve dysfunction.

FINDINGS

Sagittal T2* gradient echo images of the cervical and thoracic spine (Figs. 88.1 and 88.2, respectively) show diffuse low signal intensity involving the periphery of the cord. No intradural masses are otherwise seen. The axial T2-weighted image of the brain parenchyma (Fig. 88.3) also shows peripheral low signal intensity along the margins of the brain stem as well as low signal along the cerebellar folia.

DIAGNOSIS

Superficial siderosis.

DISCUSSION

Superficial siderosis is characterized by the deposition of hemosiderin in the leptomeninges and subpial tissues. Various symptoms are involved, including ataxia, hearing loss, myelopathy, and dementia. This results from repeated hemorrhages into the subarachnoid space. A variety of sources of bleeding have been implicated, such as aneurysms, subdural hematomas, angiomas, or tumors. In many of the cases the source of bleeding is unknown. The toxic effect of iron causes gliosis, demyelination, and nerve cell destruction leading to symptomatology. Typical MR features are low signal intensity along the pial surface of the cord and cerebellar hemispheres or cerebellum due to susceptibility artifact from hemosiderin and ferritin deposition.

BIBLIOGRAPHY

Bracchi M, Savoiardo M, Triulzi F, et al. Superficial siderosis of the CNS: MR diagnosis and clinical findings. *Am J Neuroradiol* 1993;14:227–236.

Lemmerling M, De Praeter G, Mollet P, et al. Secondary superficial siderosis of the central nervous system in a patient presenting with sensorineural hearing loss. *Neuroradiology* 1998;40:312–314.

Offenbacher H, Fazekas F, Reisecker F, et al. Superficial siderosis of the spinal cord: a rare cause of myelopathy diagnosed by MRI. *Neurology* 1991;41:1987–1989.

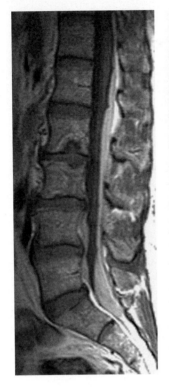

FIGURE 89.1

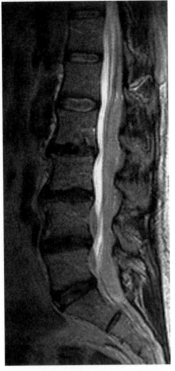

FIGURE 89.2

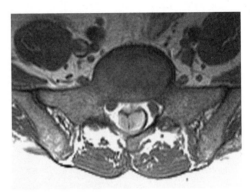

FIGURE 89.3

HISTORY

A 50-year-old with acute-onset severe low back pain while working in yard.

FINDINGS

Sagittal T1-weighted image through the lumbar spine (Fig. 89.1) shows a linear abnormal increased signal intensity following the course of the dura from L1 inferiorly through S2. This is seen both dorsally and ventrally within the thecal sac. The abnormality shows intermediate signal intensity on the fast spin echo T2-weighted image (Fig. 89.2). Axial T2-weighted image without contrast at the level of the lumbosacral junction (Fig. 89.3) demonstrates a trefoil pattern to the distal low-signal-intensity subarachnoid space, with three lobulated areas of high signal intensity around the periphery. The lesion appears intradural and laterally conforms to the dural margin.

DIAGNOSIS

Subdural hemorrhage.

DISCUSSION

Subdural hemorrhage is being recognized more commonly as a result of the use of MR. Subdural hemorrhage is capable of producing severe and irreversible neurologic deficits, and acute surgical intervention may be warranted.

Spinal subdural hematomas can have a typical configuration. As opposed to epidural hematomas, which tend to be capped by fat, subdural hematomas are located within the thecal sac and are separate from the adjacent extradural fat and the vertebral bodies posterior elements. Axial images are very useful in defining the epidural fat surrounding the thecal sac and in defining the blood relating to the interior of the sac with subdural hematomas. These may be loculated both anteriorly and posteriorly within the thecal sac. The loculation can take the form of a "Mercedes-Benz" sign, showing a trefoil configuration as in this case. Subdural hematomas should not extend out into the neural foramina; this would be more typical for an epidural hematoma. Signal characteristics can identify the abnormality as blood, but epidural and subdural hematomas are not significantly different. Acute hemorrhage can be fairly isointense on T1-weighted images but over a few days will show high signal on T1-weighted images much more typical for hemorrhage. T2 or gradient echo images are very important to obtain if there is a question of hemorrhage and will show heterogeneous low signal intensity due to the presence of deoxyhemoglobin. It is always important to search for ancillary findings, such as serpentine flow voids, which could suggest associated vascular abnormality. Spinal hematomas may be spontaneous, but multiple causative factors have been identified, such as vascular malformations, tumor, coagulopathies, trauma, prior surgery, and hypertension and anticoagulation.

BIBLIOGRAPHY

Donovan-Post MJ, Becerra JL, Madsen PW, et al. Acute spinal subdural hematoma: MR and CT findings with pathologic correlates. *Am J Neuroradiol* 1994;15:1895–1905.

Johnson PJ, Hahn F, McConnell J, et al. The importance of MRI findings for the diagnosis of nontraumatic lumbar subacute subdural haematomas. *Acta Neurochir* 1991;113:186–188.

Levy JM. Spontaneous lumbar subdural hematoma. *Am J Neuroradiol* 1990;11:780–781.

Mattle H, Sieb JP, Rohner M, et al. Nontraumatic spinal epidural and subdural hematomas. *Neurology* 1987;37:1351–1356.

Shimada Y, Sato K, Abe E, et al. Spinal subdural hematoma. *Skeletal Radiol* 1996;25:477–480.

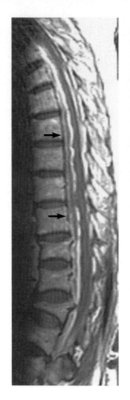
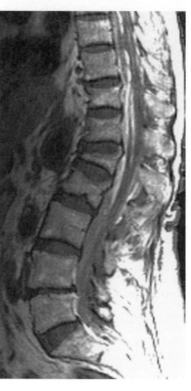

FIGURE 90.1   FIGURE 90.2

HISTORY

A 70-year-old on coumadin, with new-onset back pain and leg weakness.

FINDINGS

Sagittal T1-weighted images without contrast material of the thoracic and thoracolumbar spines (Figs. 90.1 and 90.2, respectively) show linear areas of abnormal increased signal intensity both ventral and dorsal to the thoracic cord and extending into the lumbar subarachnoid space (*arrows*). There are two linear areas of high signal separated by a line of more intermediate signal intensity, particularly noticeable in the sagittal T1 thoracic study, indicating two separate compartments of involvement. Of incidental note is multiple benign-appearing compression fractures of the thoracolumbar junction.

DIAGNOSIS

Epidural and subdural hemorrhage.

DISCUSSION

The typical clinical presentation of epidural hemorrhage is the sudden onset of back pain, which may have a radicular component. With larger collections, the signs of cord compression will develop, including long tract signs and a sensory level. The MR appearance of spinal hemorrhage can be quite variable, depending upon the location of origin and age. Acutely, the hemorrhage may be nearly isointense to cord on T1-weighted images and show mottled high signal on T2-weighted images. Gradient echo images will be helpful to highlight the mottled low signal related to deoxyhemoglobin, which is present even early on. As methemoglobin accumulates, the lesion becomes easy to define as abnormal increased signal on T1-weighted images. Axial images are often necessary to determine the site of hemorrhage, whether subdural or epidural. Epidural hemorrhage should displace the margin of the thecal sac and will extend out into the neural foramina. Subdural hemorrhage will respect the margins of the thecal sac and have a smooth lateral definition. In this case, there are two areas of involvement, both epidural and subdural. The epidural component shows up as the linear area of methemoglobin adjacent to the vertebral bodies, with a relatively low-signal separation between the linear subdural component.

BIBLIOGRAPHY

Donovan-Post MJ, Becerra JL, Madsen PW, et al. Acute spinal subdural hematoma: MR and CT findings with pathologic correlates. *Am J Neuroradiol* 1994;15:1895–1905.

Johnson PJ, Hahn F, McConnell J, et al. The importance of MRI findings for the diagnosis of nontraumatic lumbar subacute subdural haematomas. *Acta Neurochir* 1991;113:186–188.

Levy JM. Spontaneous lumbar subdural hematoma. *Am J Neuroradiol* 1990;11:780–781.

Mattle H, Sieb JP, Rohner M, et al. Nontraumatic spinal epidural and subdural hematomas. *Neurology* 1987;37:1351–1356.

Shimada Y, Sato K, Abe E, et al. Spinal subdural hematoma. *Skeletal Radiol* 1996;25:477–480.

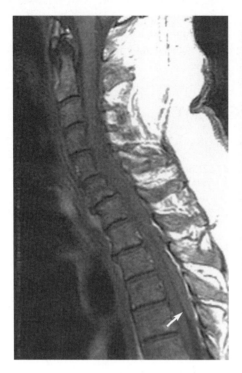
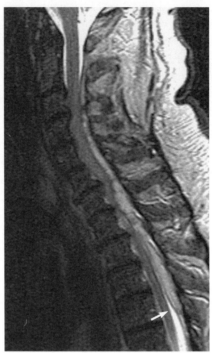

FIGURE 91.1   FIGURE 91.2

HISTORY

A 70-year-old male in the hospital for atrial fibrillation cardioversion and on heparin. The patient went to the bathroom and experienced sudden-onset quadraparesis. He was rushed to the MR suite and imaged within 1 hour of ictus.

FINDINGS

Sagittal T1-weighted image (Fig. 91.1) shows an ill-defined cervical cord that appears to be displaced anteriorly by a dorsally situated soft-tissue mass. A margin between the cord and mass is best appreciated inferiorly at the T4 level (*arrow*). The sagittal fast spin echo T2-weighted image (Fig. 91.2) better defines the slightly lobulated mass dorsal to the cord spanning C3–T4 levels. Slightly increased signal intensity is present within the cervical cord at the C4 and C5 levels. The mass itself is at a relatively obtuse angle with the dura and appears extradural in location.

DIAGNOSIS

Acute epidural hemorrhage.

DISCUSSION

Epidural spinal hemorrhage occurs most frequently in the elderly but can occur at any age. Clinically, patients develop sudden back or neck pain that may be radicular. Signs of cord compression can develop immediately or within days. Foo and Rossier reviewed the literature in 158 cases of spontaneous epidural hemorrhage and found that the postoperative return of motor function was noted in 95.3%, 87%, and 45.3% of the patients with incomplete sensorimotor, incomplete sensory but complete motor, and complete sensorimotor lesions, respectively. Complete sensorimotor recovery occurred in 41.9%, 26.1%, and 11.3% of these three groups of patients, respectively. The absence of motor or sensorimotor functions preoperatively does not necessarily indicate a poor prognosis in these patients. Occasionally, the course is a chronic undulating pattern of progressive deficits. From a clinical standpoint, the differential diagnosis is broad and includes acute disk herniation, spinal abscess, tumor, myelitis, hemorrhagic cord vascular malformation, cord infarction, and dissecting aortic aneurysm.

Spinal epidural hematomas are broadly classified into two groups: nonspontaneous and spontaneous. Nonspontaneous epidural hemorrhage may result from lumbar or C1–2 punctures, spinal anesthesia, trauma, pregnancy, bleeding diathesis, anticoagulant therapy, vascular malformations, hypertension, and neoplasms. The history can be revealing, yet it is not uncommon to consist merely of an episode of sneezing, bending, voiding, turning in bed, or mild trauma, as in this case. Spinal epidural hemorrhage can be localized or can spread anywhere along the spinal column. Blood more commonly accumulates posterolaterally. The diagnosis is suggested when the epidural lesion demonstrates classic signal properties characteristic of blood products, occurring outside of the cord and assuming a biconvex configuration with tapering superior and inferior margins.

BIBLIOGRAPHY

Avrahami E, Tadmor R, Ram Z, et al. MR demonstration of spontaneous acute epidural hematoma of the thoracic spine. *Neuroradiology* 1989;31:90–92.

Beatty RM, Winston KR. Spontaneous epidural hematoma. *J Neurosurg* 1984;61:143–148.

Bernsen PLJA, Haan J, Vielvoye GJ, et al. Spinal epidural hematoma visualized by magnetic resonance imaging. *Neuroradiology* 1988;30:280.

Foo D, Rossier AB. Preoperative neurological status in predicting surgical outcome of spinal epidural hematomas. *Surg Neurol* 1981;15:389–401.

Goldman P, Kulkarni M, MacDugall DJ, et al. Traumatic epidural hematoma of the cervical spine: diagnosis with magnetic resonance imaging. *Radiology* 1989;170-589–591.

Mattle H, Sieb JP, Rohner M, et al. Nontraumatic spinal epidural and subdural hematomas. *Neurology* 1987;37:1351–1356.

Post MJD, Seminer DS, Quencer RM. CT diagnosis of spinal epidural hematoma. *Am J Neuroradiol* 1982;3:190–192.

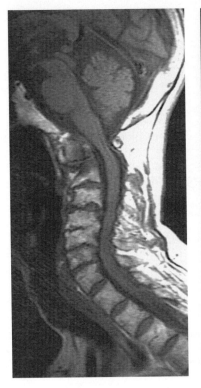

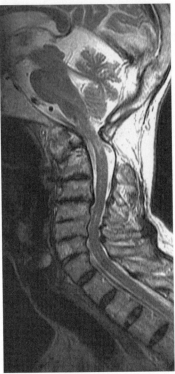

| FIGURE 92.1 | FIGURE 92.2 |

HISTORY

A 62-year-old with myelopathy and neck pain.

FINDINGS

Sagittal T1-weighted image (Fig. 92.1) shows a swan neck–like deformity of the cervical spine. The odontoid appears interrupted at its base, with a mixed signal density located posterior to the anterior arch of C1. The anterior arch of C1 itself is a semilunar area of high signal intensity. There is also moderate narrowing of the thecal sac at the C1 level due to anterior subluxation of the ring of C1 with respect to C2. There is diffuse and severe degenerative disease involving the remainder of the cervical spine. Sagittal fast spin echo T2-weighted image (Fig. 92.2) confirms the narrowed subarachnoid space at C1 as well as focal abnormal increased signal intensity within the cervical cord.

DIAGNOSIS

Os odontoideum.

DISCUSSION

Os odontoideum refers to a separate osseous structure that is located cephalad to the axis body, in the expected location of the odontoid process. The etiology of this lesion is quite debatable, with various theories postulating an embryonic, traumatic, or vascular cause. The sequela of an old odontoid fracture is a commonly proposed etiology. The importance of the anomaly is cruciate ligament incompetence and atlantoaxial instability, which leads to cord compression.

Clinical presentation is extremely variable, and patients may be asymptomatic, all the way to neck pain, transitory paretic episodes, and myelopathy. An increased incidence of os odontoideum is associated with a congenital abnormality such as Down's syndrome, Morquio's syndrome, spondy-loepiphyseal dysplasia, and Klippel-Feil anomaly. Differentiation of an os odontoideum from a type II odontoid fracture can be difficult. The fracture is more associated with a flattened and sharp, uncorticated upper margin to the axis body than a more smoothly corticated os odontoideum.

BIBLIOGRAPHY

Greene KA, Dickman CA, Marciano FF, et al. Acute axis fractures: analysis of management and outcome in 340 consecutive cases. *Spine* 1997;22:1843–1852.

Hensinger RN, Fielding JW, Hawkins RJ. Congenital anomalies of the odontoid process. *Orthop Clin North Am* 1978;9:901–912.

Schweitzer ME, Hodler J, Cervilla V, et al. Craniovertebral junction: normal anatomy with MR correlation. *Am J Roentgenol* 1992;158:1087–1090.

Smoker WR. Craniovertebral junction: normal anatomy, craniometry, and congenital anomalies. *Radiographics* 1994;14:255–277.

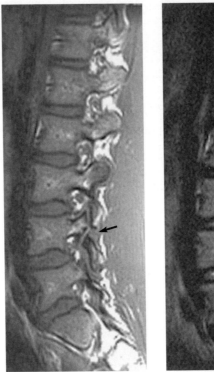

FIGURE 93.1

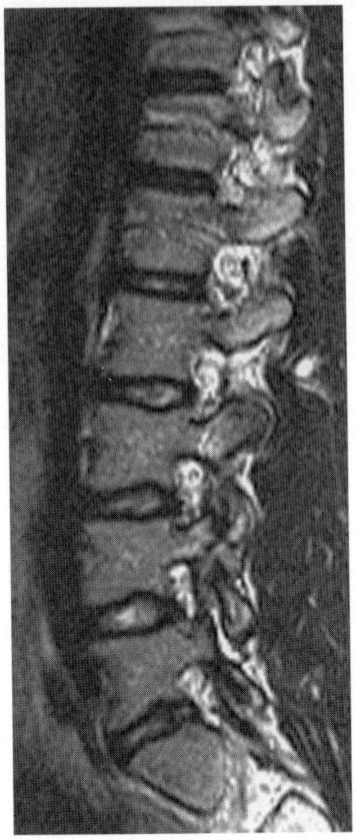

FIGURE 93.2

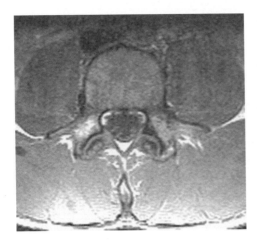

FIGURE 93.3

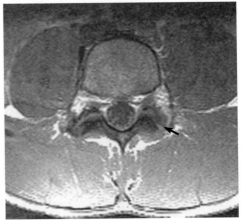

FIGURE 93.4

HISTORY

A 30-year-old with back pain.

FINDINGS

Sagittal T1-weighted image to the lumbar spine (Fig. 93.1) shows a disruption of the usual cortical low signal in-

tensity involving the left pars interarticularis at the L4 level (*arrow*). This abnormality is confirmed on the sagittal T2-

weighted image (Fig. 93.2) with slightly increased signal intensity through that region. There is also a joint effusion at L4–5, shown as high signal on the T2-weighted images. Axial T1-weighted image (Fig. 93.3) through the level of the facet at L4 shows the normal facets for comparison. Inferior to this, the axial T1-weighted image (Fig. 93.4) shows the defect on the left as an irregular area of signal intensity disrupting the cortical low signal (*arrow*).

DIAGNOSIS

L4 spondylolysis.

DISCUSSION

Because of its ability to obtain direct sagittal images free of overlapping structures and patient rotation, MR imaging is felt to be the most accurate method of diagnosing spondylolisthesis. However, the detection of spondylolysis with MR is more problematic, and it is generally agreed that plain films and CT are more reliable in this regard. However, because MR is being utilized as primarily an imaging modality for evaluating patients with low back pain and radicular symptoms, many cases of spondylolysis are imaged without correlative plain films or CT. Recognizing the MR findings associated with spondylolysis assumes even more importance. Using MR imaging, sagittal T1-weighted images are best for demonstrating the pars interarticularis due to their high signal-to-noise ratio, the depiction of the pars marrow as hyperintense, and the advantageous imaging plane for the lumbar spine. It has been shown that if the pars appears normal (i.e., contiguous normal marrow signal), then one can be certain that it is intact. However, the presence of abnormal pars signal is not specific for spondylolysis, as benign sclerosis, partial volume averaging with an adjacent degenerative facet, and osteoblastic metastases can also give this appearance. Do not forget to define any associated spondylolisthesis.

BIBLIOGRAPHY

Elster AD, Jensen KM. Computed tomography of spondylolisthesis: patterns of associated pathology. *J Comput Assist Tomogr* 1985;9:867.

Jinkins JR, Matthes JC, Sener RN, et al. Spondylolysis, spondylolisthesis, and associated nerve root entrapment in the lumbosacral spine: MR evaluation. *Am J Roentgenol* 1992;159:799.

Schiebler M, Grossman RI. Isthmic spondylolysis of the lumbar spine: MR imaging at 1.5 T. *Radiology* 1989;170:489.

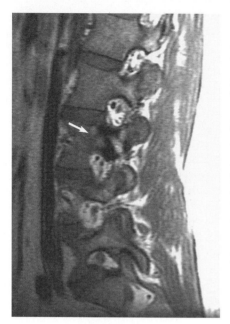

FIGURE 94.1

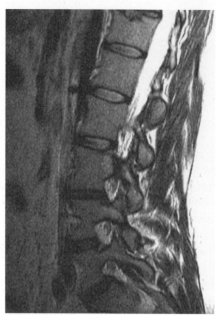

FIGURE 94.2

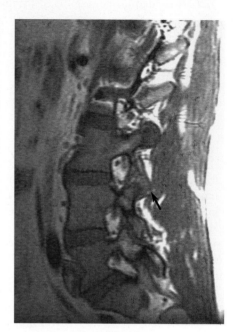

FIGURE 94.3

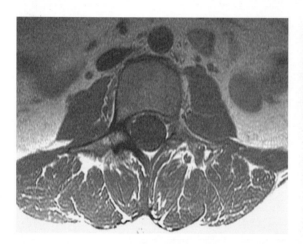

FIGURE 94.4

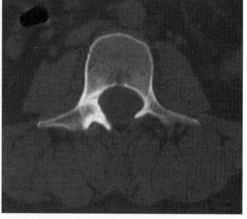

FIGURE 94.5

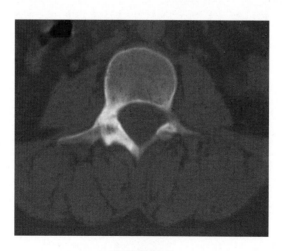

FIGURE 94.6

HISTORY

A 24-year-old with back pain.

FINDINGS

Parasagittal T1-weighted image (Fig. 94.1) through the right neural foramina shows an enlarged pedicle at the L3 level, showing mixed high and low signal intensity (*arrow*). Sagittal fast spin echo T2-weighted image also through the right foramina (Fig. 94.2) shows that the vertical low signal intensity through the pedicle is surrounded by slightly increased signal. The parasagittal T1-weighted image through the left neural foramina (Fig. 94.3) shows a very small facet at the L3 level (*arrow*). Axial T1-weighted image through the L3 level shows the low signal intensity through the right pedicle, and the very small left pedicle and small left transverse process and facet (Fig. 94.4). Two axial CT scans through the L3 level (Figs. 94.5 94.6) show bony sclerosis of the pedicle, which has a lucency extending transversely through the pedicle. There is also confirmation of the hypoplastic left facet and pedicle.

DIAGNOSIS

Right L3 pars interarticularis fracture with sclerosis, and left hypoplastic facet.

DISCUSSION

Spondylolysis is a defect in the pars interarticularis, which may be found in 3% to 10% of the general population. The most universally accepted hypothesis is that these pars defects result from stress fractures due to repeated trauma. Most likely, there are other factors than simply mechanical trauma related to upright gait, because hereditary factors do appear to predispose to the development of pars interarticularis defects. The L5 vertebra is the most commonly affected by spondylolysis, with most of these defects at L5 being bilateral. Spondylolysis by itself may produce little symptomatology. However, it may predispose to additional abnormalities, such as degenerative facet disease, compression, or compromise of the exiting nerve root within the neural foramen and spondylolisthesis. Imaging of pars defects on MR can be problematic, since low signal intensity on the T1-weighted images may simply reflect the opposition of adjacent cortical bone within the pars interarticularis. However, when this low signal is intervened by well-defined increased signal on the T2, a more definitive diagnosis of a pars defect can be identified. Of course, in more blatant lysis, there is enough separation of the fragments to allow easy diagnosis.

In this example, the right-sided defect in the pars is difficult to identify on MR, although the abnormal bony sclerosis is identified as areas of low signal intensity. The axial images do allow the diagnosis of the fracture site. The cause of the right defect is the hypoplastic facet that, occurring on the left, alters the biomechanics at that level. CT is confirmatory, showing not only the bony ebernation of the pedicle in the adjacent bone, but the fracture site itself.

BIBLIOGRAPHY

Johnson WJ, Farnum GN, Latchaw RE, et al. MR imaging of the pars interarticularis. *Am J Roentgenol* 1989;152:327.
Ulmer JL, Elster AD, Mathews VP, et al. Lumbar spondylolysis: reactive marrow changes seen in adjacent pedicles on MR images. *Am J Roentgenol* 1995;169:429.
Ulmer JL, Elster AD, Mathews VP, et al. Distinction between degenerative and isthmic spondylolisthesis on sagittal MR images: importance of increased anteroposterior diameter of the spinal canal ("wide canal sign"). *Am J Roentgenol* 1994;163:411.

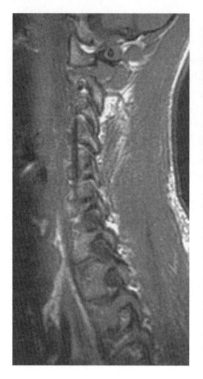

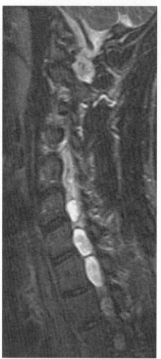

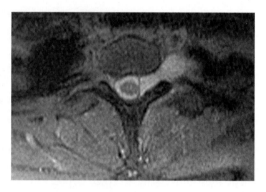

| FIGURE 95.1 | FIGURE 95.2 | FIGURE 95.3 |

HISTORY

A 40-year-old with left arm weakness and a history of trauma.

FINDINGS

Sagittal T1-weighted image through the left neural foramina (Fig. 95.1) shows low signal intensity within the foramina at the C6, C7, and T1 levels. The abnormal signal is confirmed on the left parasagittal T2-weighted image (Fig. 95.2), showing rounded areas of CSF signal intensity along the lateral margin of the thecal sac. The abnormality is better identified on the axial gradient echo image (Fig. 95.3) through the C7–T1 levels with CSF signal intensity extending out into the left neural foramen, as well as showing a dural margin that is straightened along the left lateral aspect of the thecal sac.

DIAGNOSIS

Pseudomeningoceles from traumatic cervical root avulsion.

DISCUSSION

Although MR imaging can define the pseudomeningoceles associated with traumatic root avulsion, myelography and CT myelography remain the gold standard. Nearly 100% of root evulsions have been detected using CT/CT myelography in contrast to MR imaging. Volle et al. found the sensitivities of cervical myelography, CT myelography, and MR to be 100%, 45%, and 6%, respectively, for nerve root avulsions. Evaluation of these patients not only showed a level of avulsion but also documented overall size and morphology of the associated pseudomeningoceles. MR imaging has difficulty, since the pseudomeningocele can occur without a root avulsion and root avulsions may occur without pseudomeningoceles. High-resolution imaging, potentially with steady-state sequences and three-dimensional imaging, may allow evaluation of the exiting or entering rootlets and more specifically define sites of avulsion.

BIBLIOGRAPHY

Carvalho GA, Nikkhah G, Matthies C, et al. Diagnosis of root avulsions in traumatic brachial plexus injuries: value of computerized tomography myelography and magnetic resonance imaging. *J Neurosurg* 1997;86:69–76.

Gasparotti R, Ferraresi S, Pinelli L, et al. Three-dimensional MR myelography of traumatic injuries of the brachial plexus. *Am J Neuroradiol* 1997;18:1733–1742.

Hashimoto T, Mitomo M, Hirabuki N, et al. Nerve root avulsion of birth palsy: comparison of myelography with CT myelography and somatosensory evoked potential. *Radiology* 1991;178:841–845.

Hayashi N, Yamamoto S, Okubo T, et al. Avulsion injury of cervical nerve roots: enhanced intradural nerve roots at MR imaging. *Radiology* 1998;206:817–822.

Volle E, Assheuer J, Hedd J, et al. Radicular evulsion resulting from spinal injury: assessment of diagnostic modalities. *Neuroradiology* 1992;34:235.

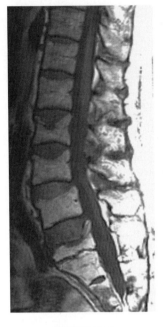

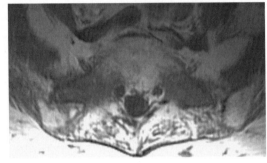

FIGURE 96.1   **FIGURE 96.2**

HISTORY

A 75-year-old female with low back pain.

FINDINGS

Sagittal T1-weighted image through the lumbar spine (Fig. 96.1) shows old compression fractures at the L2, L3, and L5 levels. There is mild posterior bony retropulsion at L5. Linear low signal intensity is seen within the midportion of the S2 body. Axial T1-weighted image (Fig. 96-2) demonstrates abnormal low signal intensity involving the sacral ala bilaterally in a symmetric fashion. There is no evidence of soft-tissue extension beyond the bony cortical margins.

DIAGNOSIS

Sacral insufficiency fracture.

DISCUSSION

Osteoporosis and radiation therapy are the main predisposing factors for insufficiency fractures of the pelvis. These abnormalities may be difficult to diagnose for several reasons. The findings on the plain films are easily overlooked and subtle. The primary finding is often sclerosis that is related to trabecular compression. The fractures also run vertically along the sacral ala and parallel to the sacroiliac joints. MR can be sensitive to detecting early medullary edema and can be very helpful in defining the fracture sites. Axial T1- and T2-weighted images are useful for eliminating any soft-tissue component, which would minimize the suspicion for metastatic infiltration. Often a discrete fracture line may not be defined on MR. Injection of contrast with fat-suppressed T1-weighted techniques also can help delineate a fracture site. Overall, the location of the edema on T2-weighted images, parallel to the SI joint, and the presence of a fracture line are virtually diagnostic of an insufficiency fracture. In the presence of edema without a fracture line, follow-up would be recommended.

BIBLIOGRAPHY

Baker RJJ, Siegel A. Sacral insufficiency fracture: half of an "H." *Clin Nucl Med* 1994;19:1106–1107.

Dasgupta B, Shah N, Brown H, et al. Sacral insufficiency fractures: an unsuspected cause of low back pain. *Br J Rheumatol* 1998;37:789–793.

Grangier C, Garcia J, Howarth NR, et al. Role of MRI in the diagnosis of insufficiency fractures of the sacrum and acetabular roof. *Skeletal Radiol* 1997;26:517–524.

Grasland A, Pouchot J, Mathieu A, et al. Sacral insufficiency fractures: an easily overlooked cause of back pain in elderly women. *Arch Intern Med* 1996;156:668–674.

Peh WC, Khong PL, Yin Y, et al. Imaging of pelvic insufficiency fractures. *Radiographics* 1996;16:335–348.

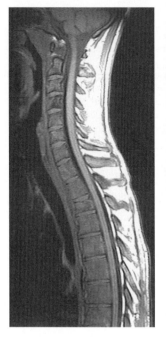

FIGURE 97.1

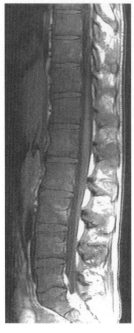

FIGURE 97.2

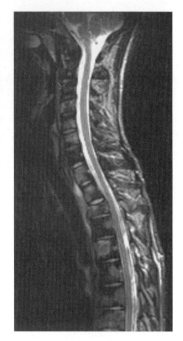

FIGURE 97.3

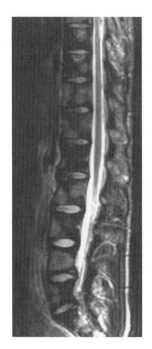

FIGURE 97.4

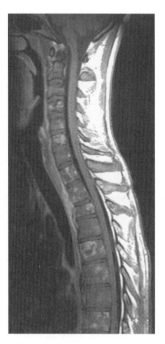

FIGURE 97.5

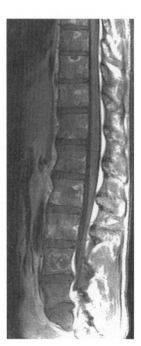

FIGURE 97.6

HISTORY

A 19-year-old with upper back pain.

FINDINGS

Sagittal T1-weighted images of the axial skeleton (Figs. 97.1 and 97.2) show diffusely abnormal low signal intensity throughout all the visualized vertebral bodies and posterior elements. There is moderate collapse of the T3 vertebral body with no significant posterior retropulsion. There is no evidence of epidural soft-tissue mass and no evidence of cord compression. Sagittal fast spin echo T2-weighted images (Figs. 97.3 and 97.4) show mottled abnormal increased and decreased signal intensity from the vertebral bodies and posterior elements. Following contrast administration, the sagittal T1-weighted images (Figs. 97.5 and 97.6) demonstrate mottled and abnormal enhancement within multiple vertebral bodies, sparing the intravertebral disk. No abnormal intradural or intramedullary enhancement is seen.

DIAGNOSIS

Pathologic compression fracture due to non-Hodgkin's lymphoma.

DISCUSSION

Metastatic disease to the spine is by far the most common type of extradural tumor. Because of its high-contrast sensitivity and spatial resolution, MR imaging is the examination of choice in the detection of osseous metastases. In addition, MR provides accurate assessment of the effects of metastatic disease on the cord, conus medullaris, and thecal sac in a much earlier time frame than can be depicted on plain radiography. MR depicts tumor replacement of the normal high-signal fatty marrow on T1-weighted images as focal or diffuse areas of low signal intensity. Because many metastatic tumors enhance, the routine use of contrast-enhanced studies alone is not recommended for the identification of bony metastatic disease because the contrast between metastases and normal marrow fat is diminished. Contrast is useful if there is any question of leptomeningeal metastatic disease and may be helpful with fat suppression for extent of epidural disease. T2-weighted images are generally not required in a screening study for patients suspected of having metastases. However, in evaluating patients with low marrow signal on T1-weighted images related to other nonneoplastic causes, contrast enhancement, T2-weighted imaging, or short inversion time inversion-recovery (STIR) imaging may be useful. In one retrospective study of 58 patients, the authors concluded that MR was the examination of choice for the evaluation of suspected metastases to the spine (Fig. 97.1). A prospective study of 70 patients with known or suspected spinal involvement by malignancy demonstrated sensitivities and specificities of 0.92 and 0.90, respectively, for MR evaluation of extradural masses causing cord compression (Fig. 97.2). The advantages of MR include (a) the avoidance of the complications of thecal puncture in patients with complete block or bleeding dyscrasias, (b) the ability to image patients who could not tolerate a C1–2 puncture, (c) demonstration of mild vertebral body or epidural disease, and (d) imaging areas between subarachnoid blocks.

Although diffuse osseous metastases can appear as homogeneous diffuse low marrow signal on T1-weighted images, this appearance is not specific. Other marrow replacement disorders such as myelofibrosis, myeloproliferative syndromes, lymphoma, leukemia, and multiple myeloma may have this appearance. Nonneoplastic entities such as marrow reconversion secondary to chronic anemias, iron overload states, and sclerosis secondary to chronic renal disease will also show abnormal low signal.

BIBLIOGRAPHY

Carmody RF, Yang PJ, Seeley GW, et al. Spinal cord compression due to metastatic disease: diagnosis with MR imaging versus myelography. *Radiology* 1989;173:225.

Smolen WR, Godersky JC, Knutzon RK, et al. The role of MR imaging in evaluating metastatic spinal disease. *Am J Neuroradiol* 1987;8:901.

Sze G, Abramson A, Krol G, et al. Gadolinium-DTPA: malignant extradural spinal tumors. *Radiology* 1988;67:217.

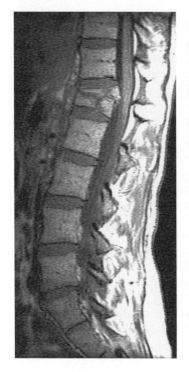

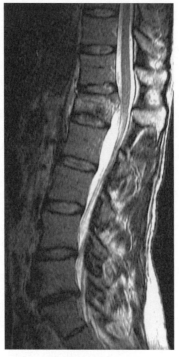

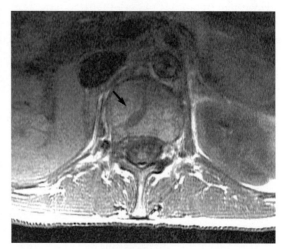

FIGURE 98.1

FIGURE 98.2

FIGURE 98.3

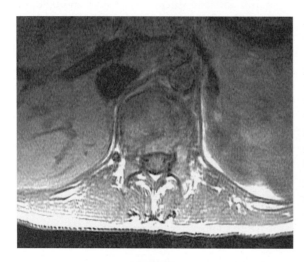

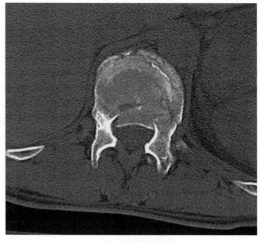

FIGURE 98.4

FIGURE 98.5

HISTORY

A 52-year-old who fell from a ladder.

FINDINGS

Sagittal T1-weighted image (Fig. 98.1) shows moderate loss of height and anterior wedging of the L1 vertebral body. There is posterior retropulsion of the posterior superior as-pect of the vertebral body that effaces the anterior aspect of the thecal sac and just touches the conus. There is a Y-shaped low signal intensity within the vertebral body. Sagittal fast spin echo T2-weighted image (Fig. 98.2) also demonstrates the posterior retropulsion without conus compromise. Axial T1-weighted images through the L1 body (Figs. 98.3 and 98.4) show an oblique fracture line extending through the right side of the vertebral body (*arrow*), as well as the posteriorly retropulsed posterior superior end plate. Axial CT image through the retropulsed level (Fig. 98.5) shows the thecal sac narrowing on the order of 40% by the bony fragment.

DIAGNOSIS

L1 burst fracture.

DISCUSSION

The thoracolumbar junction is a common site for injuries to the spine because of the transition from the relatively immobile thoracic segment to the mobile lumbar segment. Biomechanical studies have led to the concept of three spinal columns that are important for stability: anterior, middle, and posterior columns. The anterior column extends from the anterior longitudinal ligament to the midportion of the vertebral body. The middle column extends from the mid vertebral body posteriorly to include the posterior longitudinal ligament. The posterior column includes all bony and soft-tissue elements dorsal to the posterior longitudinal ligament. Considering the various pathomechanics of spine injuries (flexion, extension, distraction, compression, shearing, and rotation) in combination with this three-column concept, spinal injuries can be classified. A compression fracture is the result of failure of the anterior column in flexion. A burst fracture is a result of failure of the anterior and middle columns in compression. A Chance fracture is a result of failure of the middle and posterior columns in distraction. A fracture dislocation is a result of failure of all three columns under various types of stress. In general, fractures that involve the middle column are considered unstable, whereas fractures that spare the middle column are considered stable.

The main technique for evaluation of spinal column injuries is conventional radiography, which detects fractures and dislocations. Fractures that are visible on plain films may be further evaluated with CT or conventional tomography. CT remains the method of choice for the detection of retropulsed bony fragments and for the demonstration of fractures of the posterior elements.

The advantages of MR in the evaluation of spinal trauma include its noninvasiveness and its superb rendition of the spinal canal contents and paraspinal soft tissue. T1- and T2-weighted images are useful in evaluating the trauma patient. Intramedullary and ligamentous abnormalities are often best seen on the T2-weighted spin echo images. At present, contrast medium has little role in the evaluation of trauma. Thin-section gradient echo images may be optimal for evaluation of the facet joints.

Although CT is more sensitive than MR for detecting bony abnormalities, MR is often superior for evaluating soft-tissue structures. In particular, the spinal ligaments show focal discontinuity on T1-weighted images and areas of increased signal intensity on T2-weighted images. The anterior and posterior longitudinal, flaval, interspinous, and supraspinous ligaments can all be evaluated, often most favorably in the sagittal plane. Sagittal and axial images can define retropulsed bony fragments and narrowing of the spinal canal. MR excels at noninvasively imaging the cord and any compression from bony fragments. MR appears to be less sensitive than CT in detecting fractures involving the posterior elements.

BIBLIOGRAPHY

Blumenkopf B, Juneau-PA II. Magnetic resonance imaging (MRI) of thoracolumbar fractures. *J Spinal Disord* 1988;1:144–150.

Brightman RP, Miller CA, Rea GL, et al. Magnetic resonance imaging of trauma to the thoracic and lumbar spine: the importance of the posterior longitudinal ligament. *Spine* 1992;17:541–550.

Denis F. The three column spine and its significance in the classification of acute thoracolumbar spine injuries. *Spine* 1983;8:817.

Smith WS, Kaufer H. Patterns and mechanisms of lumbar injuries associated with lap seat belts. *J Bone Joint Surg Am* 1969;52:239.

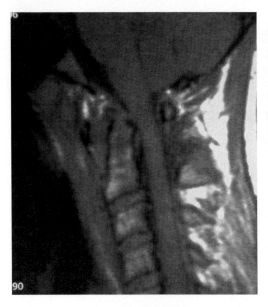

FIGURE 99.1

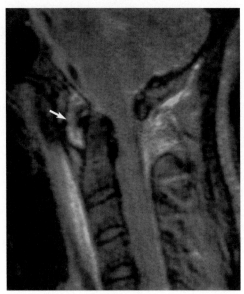

FIGURE 99.2

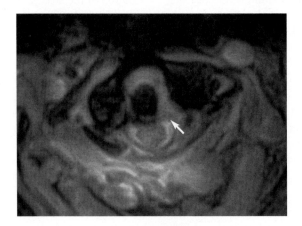

FIGURE 99.3

HISTORY

A 30-year-old following a motor vehicle accident.

FINDINGS

Sagittal T1-weighted image through the craniovertebral junction (Fig. 99.1) shows widening of the atlantodental interval. Abnormal increased signal is noted within the predental space. There is narrowing of the subarachnoid space between the posterior arch of C1 and the posterior margin of the odontoid. Sagittal fast spin echo T2-weighted image (Fig. 99.2) confirms the abnormal signal within the preden-

tal space (*arrow*), as well as high-signal-intensity edema within the prevertebral regions spanning C2–4. Abnormal increased signal is also present within the posterior ligamentous complex between the posterior arch of C1 and C2. There is widening of the posterior margins of C1 and C2 as well. Axial gradient echo image through the C1 level (Fig. 99.3) shows the increased atlantodental interval with increased signal intensity. Increased signal is also seen dorsally within the soft tissues along the posterior arch of C1. The transverse ligament is identified on the right as low signal intensity but shows abnormal high signal intensity on the left (*arrow*).

DIAGNOSIS

Transverse ligament disruption.

DISCUSSION

Injuries involving the transverse atlantal ligament may be classified into two types, type I and type II, depending upon the extent of injury to the ligaments and bone involved, as described by Dickman et al. Disruptions within the substance of the transverse ligament are defined at type I. These are incapable of healing and should be treated with early surgery for internal fixation. Type II lesions involve an injury disconnecting the tubercle and the insertion of the transverse ligament from the C1 lateral mass. This is not an injury within the substance of the ligament itself. In 74% of cases in one series, these healed with nonoperative treatment using external immobilization.

Plain radiographs alone are inadequate to define the morphologic pattern of injury to the transverse ligament but may be used as a screening tool to detect possible abnormality. The normal relationship of C1 lateral masses on an open-mouth view or a normal atlantodental interval on a lateral plain film does not exclude injury to the transverse ligament. Some authors do not advocate flexion and extension views with extensive fractures of C1 and C2, even if the atlantodental interval is normal on static radiographs because of the risk of neurologic injury. In that setting, with a lack of functional evaluation, CT and MR are mandatory. CT and MR are complementary, with CT demonstrating the bone structure and MR showing the soft-tissue anatomy. The normal transverse ligament is a homogenous low signal on the gradient echo axial images, with disruption showing anatomic discontinuity and high signal intensity.

BIBLIOGRAPHY

Dickman CA, Greene KA, Sonntag VK. Injuries involving the transverse atlantal ligament: classification and treatment guidelines based upon experience with 39 injuries. *Neurosurgery* 1996;38:44–50.

Findlay JM. Injuries involving the transverse atlantal ligament: classification and treatment guidelines based upon experience with 39 injuries. *Neurosurgery* 1996;39:210.

Greene KA, Dickman CA, Marciano FF, et al. Transverse atlantal ligament disruption associated with odontoid fractures. *Spine* 1994;19:2307–2314.

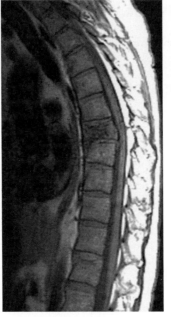

FIGURE 100.1   **FIGURE 100.2**

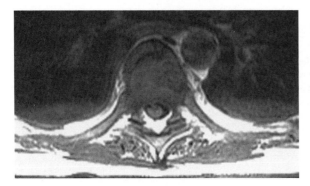

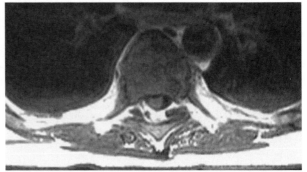

FIGURE 100.3   **FIGURE 100.4**

HISTORY

A 39-year-old paraplegic 3 years after a motor vehicle accident, with increasing thoracic pain.

FINDINGS

Sagittal T1-weighted image through the thoracic spine (Fig. 100.1) shows loss of height and abnormal signal intensity within the T6 vertebral body. There is slight posterior retropulsion of the inferior posterior aspect of the body that mildly effaces the intrathecal sac. Sagittal fast spin echo T2-weighted image (Fig. 100.2) shows the mild effacement of the sac interiorly by the posterior bony retropulsion. The focal area of abnormally increased signal is seen within the thoracic cord at this level. Axial T1-weighted images through the vertebral body and intravertebral disk at the level below (Figs. 100.3 and 100.4) shows small central protrusion of the disk that mildly faces the anterior cord. Linear lucency is seen extending through the vertebral body itself, reflecting the fracture site.

DIAGNOSIS

T6 burst fracture, with cystic myelomalacia and disk herniation.

DISCUSSION

Evaluation of acute spinal trauma continues to rely on plain film and CT examination. MR can assess the cord directly and its relationship to the surrounding structures. Cord edema and hemorrhage can easily be detected in the acutely traumatized spinal cord. Cord edema can cause focal enlargement of the cord and prolongs T1 and T2 due to increased water content. This is usually best seen on T2-weighted images as an area of increased signal intensity. Prognostically, it may be helpful to distinguish an edematous cord from a hemorrhagic contusion because the former has a better prognosis. Cord transection represents the most severe form of cord injury and is usually seen as a decreased or heterogeneous cord signal, or frank discontinuity of the cord.

In patients who have neurologic deficits after injury to the spinal cord, new symptoms can be seen at a considerable period after the time of injury. This entity has been termed *posttraumatic progressive myelopathy*. It may be caused by the development of intramedullary cysts (syringohydromyelia) or to noncystic lesions, such as myelomalacia. Cysts may occur above or below the site of injury. It is important to distinguish these causes, since symptoms due to syringomyelia may be reduced after surgical shunting.

MR imaging can usually differentiate between posttraumatic cysts and myelomalacia. On T1-weighted images, both cysts and myelomalacia are low in signal compared with the spinal cord (similar to CSF). On intermediate (proton density) or fluid attenuated inversion recovery (FLAIR) images, a syrinx continues to show low signal, but myelomalacia becomes isointense or slightly hyperintense with respect to the cord. T2-weighted images show high signal for both entities. A cyst will demonstrate a sharper interface with the spinal cord than will myelomalacia.

BIBLIOGRAPHY

Falcone S, Quencer RM, Green BA, et al. Progressive posttraumatic myelomalacic myelopathy: imaging and clinical features. *Am J Neuroradiol* 1994;15:747–754.

Gebarski SS, Maynard FW, Gabrielsen TO, et al. Posttraumatic progressive myelopathy: clinical and radiologic correlation employing MR imaging, delayed CT metrizamide myelography, and intraoperative sonography. *Radiology* 1985;157:379–385.

Jinkins JR, Reddy S, Leite CC, et al. MR of parenchymal spinal cord signal change as a sign of active advancement in clinically progressive posttraumatic syringomyelia. *Am J Neuroradiol* 1998;19:177–182.

Milhorat TH, Johnson WD, Miller JI, et al. Surgical treatment of syringomyelia based on magnetic resonance imaging criteria. *Neurosurgery* 1992;31:231–244.

Quencer RM, El Gammal T, Cohen G. Syringomyelia associated with intradural, extramedullary masses of the spinal canal. *Am J Neuroradiol* 1986;7:143–148.

Quencer RM, Sheldon JJ, Post MJD, et al. MRI of the chronically injured cervical spinal cord. *Am J Neuroradiol* 1986;7:457–464.

Sherman JL, Barkovich AJ, Citrin CA. The MR appearance of syringomyelia: new observations. *Am J Neuroradiol* 1986;7:985–995.

Yamashita Y, Takahashi M, Matsuno Y, et al. Chronic injuries of the spinal cord: assessment with MR imaging. *Radiology* 1990;175:849–854.

SUBJECT INDEX

Page numbers followed by an f refer to figures.